## DATE DUE

| | |
|---|---|
| DEC - 6 1997 | |
| OCT 1 6 1998 | |
| NOV 1 4 2001 | |
| Rgon 10374205 | |
| | |
| | |
| | |
| | |
| | |
| | |
| | |
| | |
| | |
| | |
| | |
| | |
| | |

# NURSING THEORIES AND QUALITY OF CARE

# Nursing Theories and Quality of Care

**HUGH P. McKENNA**
*School of Health Sciences*
*University of Ulster*

# Avebury

Aldershot · Brookfield USA · Hong Kong · Singapore · Sydney

© H. P. McKenna 1994

Published by
Avebury
Ashgate Publishing Limited
Gower House
Croft Road
Aldershot
Hants GU11 3HR
England

Ashgate Publishing Company
Old Post Road
Brookfield
Vermont 05036
USA

**British Library Cataloguing in Publication Data**

McKenna, P. Hugh
    Nursing Theories and Quality of Care. -
    (Developments in Nursing & Health Care
    Series)
    I. Title  II. Series
    610.73
ISBN 1 85628 670 3

**Library of Congress Cataloging-in-Publication Data**

McKenna, Hugh P., 1954–
    Nursing theories and quality of care / Hugh P. McKenna.
        p.   cm. -- (Developments in nursing and health care : 1)
    Includes bibliographical references.
    ISBN 1-85628-670-3 : $59.95 (est.)
    1. Psychiatric nursing--Philosophy--Case studies. 2. Nursing
    models--Evaluation--Case studies. 3. Psychiatric nursing-
    -Evaluation--Case studies. I. Title. II. Series.
    [DNLM: 1. Psychiatric Nursing. 2. Models, Nursing. 3. Quality of
    Health Care--standards. WY 160 M478n 1994]
    RC440.M33    1994
    610.73'68--dc20
    DNLM/DLC
    for Library of Congress                                    94-6399
                                                                CIP

Printed and Bound in Great Britain by
Athenaeum Press Ltd, Newcastle upon Tyne.

# Contents

# Figures and tables

vii

ix

# Acknowledgements

First and foremost, my sincere thanks are due to the patients and staff whose help and co-operation enabled me to undertake this research. I am also indebted to Dr K. Parahoo and Professor J.R.P. Boore without whose help the thesis could not have been completed. I also wish to thank those academics who allowed me to use their research instruments and those who assisted me in determining content validity for some of the tools. Last but not least, I wish to sincerely thank my wife Tricia and my children Gowain and Saoirse for often having to put up with an absentee husband and father; also my mother whose prayers must have contributed to the completion of the study.

# Summary

This is a two part research study concerning the selection of a nursing model for long-stay psychiatric care, and evaluation of the effects of the selected model on quality of care. For part one, a survey approach was used. Three research instruments were devised from the literature and presented to ninety five ward managers from Northern Ireland's long-stay psychiatric wards. The 'theoretical bases instrument' was composed of concise summaries of the four main theoretical underpinnings for nursing models. Responses indicated that 68% favoured Behavioural theory, 20% Interactional theory, 9% Developmental theory and 3% Systems theory.

Each nursing model also incorporates specific views on four value-laden components. These are, Nursing, Person, Health, and Environment. These 'essential elements' were extracted from nineteen of the most popular nursing models to formulate a 'model matrix'. Using a modified version of the 'Delphi technique' this instrument was presented in two rounds to all the research respondents. Of the 95 respondents 61% selected the 'Human Needs' model (HNM) of Minshull et al (1986). A semi-structured interview schedule completed with all the respondents elicited information on their views on nursing models. Results showed that 61% held positive opinions about nursing models, 23% held negative opinions, while 14% and 2% gave undecided or indifferent opinions respectively.

In part two of the study an action research approach was used to implement the HNM on a long-stay psychiatric ward. Within a broader quasi-experimental design selected quality of care indicators were appraised before and after the implementation of the model. These dependent variables were also monitored on a control ward. Data were collected on both wards at one pretest and two posttest points using a triangulation of mostly quantitative research methods. The research instruments used emanated from the literature and the field work lasted nearly nine months. Results indicated that on the experimental ward there were statistically significant improvements in 'psychiatric monitor', patients' and staffs' perception of ward atmosphere, patient satisfaction, staffs' views about nursing models, and patient dependency levels. Positive change was also noted in other dependent variables not amenable to statistical analysis. No significant change was noted in medication patterns, nurse satisfaction levels and nurses' perception of patients' behaviour. However the findings from this study must be examined in the light of competing explanations and the attempts by the researcher to control for them.

# Part 1
## SELECTING AN APPROPRIATE NURSING MODEL

# 1 Introduction

**Background to the study**

The knowledge base of a profession is normally expressed in the form of concepts, models and theories. In the United Kingdom (UK) some nurses are currently developing a body of knowledge incorporating these elements. American literature on this subject dates from the early 1950s and several books by British authors have been published (Roper et al, 1985; Chapman, 1985; Aggleton and Chalmers, 1986; Kershaw and Savage, 1986; Pearson and Vaughan, 1986; Salvage and Kershaw, 1990; Wright, 1986,1990; Fraser, 1990; Walsh, 1991). These publications have been accompanied by workshops and conferences throughout the UK.

This relatively recent popularity has also been reinforced by the United Kingdom Central Council for Nursing, Midwifery and Health Visiting, which has voiced its support for nursing models (Girot, 1990). Kershaw (1990) states that: "The D.H.S.S. 'Strategy for Nursing' takes as implicit that model based practice occurs." (p.36). Cash (1990) goes further by saying that: " Models are now an explicit part of the curricula for registered nurses." (p.249).

According to Pearson (1986), a move toward model-based practice is the most important target for change within nursing. Castledine (1986), believes that the implementation of a nursing model leads to better nursing care and more reliable and critical observation by the nurse.

This study evolved from personal experience in clinical nursing practice. As a charge nurse in an acute psychiatric unit I was actively involved in considering the implementation of a model of nursing. After much discussion, reading and reflection I was aware of two problems facing the clinician:

3

1    How do practising nurses select a nursing model that is appropriate for their patient care group?

2    How do practising nurses know if the selected model will be effective in improving the quality of patient care?

Unfortunately the literature identified little or no research to help nurses answer these questions.

Therefore this study is a two part investigation. The first part is concerned with the selection by ward managers of an appropriate nursing model for the care of long-stay psychiatric patients and their opinions towards models. The second part involves appraising how the quality of care on a long-stay psychiatric ward is affected by the implementation of the selected model.

*Justification for the study*

It would be naive to believe that the forty or more nursing models now available are all inherently good. Furthermore, Ellis (1982) points out that nursing as a profession has much to lose by jumping on another bandwagon or embracing another fad.

Some writers would argue that one model is better than another or that one can lend itself to use in all nursing situations. Indeed different nurse theorists assert that their particular conceptual framework is the best. Wright (1986) also warns of the difficulties arising if one model is imposed across a broad range of hospital wards. Unfortunately the literature shows that this is not an uncommon occurrence. Similarly, how patients are assessed and how their care is planned, implemented and evaluated is determined to a large extent by the particular nursing model in use.

The literature suggests that the type of patient and the type of patient care setting are important factors to consider when selecting a nursing model. This study focused on long-stay psychiatric patients. This group was selected because Brooking (1986) found that they have been neglected by most nurse researchers. Moreover, most long-stay patients can respond to questions and are on the same ward over a long period; for research purposes these factors give them an advantage over many of those patients in psychogeriatric or acute admission wards.

It was decided that the ward sisters/charge nurses should be involved in the selection of an appropriate nursing model. A comprehensive review of many research studies by Alexander and Orton (1988) concluded that the ward sister/charge nurse:

...emerged as the key figure within the organization and the ward team, managing, coordinating and giving care, creating the ward climate...it is mainly this grade of nurse who initiates or blocks changes in nursing practice." (p.38).

Therefore, in part one of this study, ward managers in Northern Ireland were involved in selecting what they believed to be an appropriate nursing model for long-stay psychiatric patient care and in giving their opinions regarding nursing models.

# 2 Literature review: non-nursing models

## The use of models in mental health

Models are conceptual tools or devices that can be used by an individual or group to understand and place more complex phenomena in perspective. All models are made up of concepts that are related in some way. They help individuals to organize their thinking about everyday events and then to transfer their thinking into practice with order and effectiveness (Wright, 1986).

Riehl and Roy (1974) emphasize that models have been employed in all fields of scientific enquiry. Their function is the same despite professional origin. They seek to clarify and explain. Mathematicians have used models for this purpose for thousands of years. Physics, the most basic of human sciences can trace its application of models back to the Greek Atomists. In biology, Watson and Crick who discovered the structure of D.N.A., postponed celebrations and publication until after they had constructed the double helix model. Models are also used extensively in the social sciences of psychology, sociology and public relations (Riehl and Roy, 1974).

Whether they are aware of it or not the care and treatment of patients is influenced by whatever model the practitioner decides to use (Botha, 1989). Currently four main non-nursing conceptual frameworks are recognized as having had an impact on the delivery of mental health care. They are used by contemporary mental health practitioners, sometimes exclusively and competing, sometimes hand in hand (Clare, 1976). Each one attempts to explain psychiatric disorders and acts as a basis for professional practice. They are:

The medical model;
The psychotherapeutic model;

6

The behavioural model;
The sociotherapeutic model.

*The medical model*

The medical model of psychiatry emphasizes that mental disorders are illnesses (not unlike physical illnesses), caused by genetic, biochemical, traumatic or pathological disturbances and may be treated by chemotherapy, electrotherapy or sometimes psychosurgery. Social and psychological factors have little currency within this basic precept. However, in some areas of psychiatry the influences of these factors are considered, albeit in a subordinate relationship to physical changes in the organism (Stuart and Sundeen, 1983).

*Nursing and the medical model*   The development of an educational system for mental nurses in the United Kingdom occurred against the background of the medicalization of psychiatry. General hospital practices, with their foundations firmly embedded in the medical model, were applied throughout the psychiatric services. Attendants became nurses, lunatics became patients, asylums became hospitals and matrons and assistant matrons from general hospitals were recruited to lead the nursing teams (Nolan, 1985). Given this background it is not surprising that the medical model became prominent in psychiatric nursing.

Within the medical model psychiatric nurses were restricted from developing therapeutic relationships with patients as this was reserved for the medical staff (Dienemann, 1976). Psychiatrists believed that their work should not be tampered with by others, especially 'lesser others' (Goffman, 1961). The servile 'hand maiden' image of nursing is believed by some British nurse researchers to be due to the tenacious reliance on the medical model (Towell, 1975; Cormack, 1981). Chapman (1985) maintains that the medical model does not allow for independent nursing action and that armed with this model the nurse is ill equipped to envisage and help the patient as a whole person.

Although the medical frame of reference is undergoing critical examination, there is evidence from Scotland that it remains a major influence in the delivery of mental health nursing (Barker, 1990). This problem is not unique to psychiatric care nor to the United Kingdom. Stevens (1979), an American author believes that all branches of nursing are in a state of flux, trying to decide whether to relate to or seek independence from, the medical model.

Traditional subordination to physicians and the carrying out of their orders, may remain with nursing for some time to come. Meanwhile, Altschul (1981) emphasized

7

that the dislike of the medical model by psychiatric nurses led them to take an interest in models contributed by other disciplines.

## The psychotherapeutic model

Sigmund Freud (1856-1939) has been referred to as the father of psychotherapy. His theoretical assumptions, a subject of much criticism, have nevertheless influenced many psychological therapies carried out by some psychiatric nurses today. Freud's background was clearly medically based and in the early part of his career he openly subscribed to the medical model (Siegler and Osmond, 1974). Some of his followers departed from orthodox Freudian theory and formed the Neo-Freudians. They put forward the idea of Interpersonal Psychotherapy, an important development for psychiatric nursing.

*Nurses' involvement in psychotherapy*  Nurse involvement in psychotherapy gained momentum in the United States in the late 1940's and early 1950's and the idea of psychotherapeutic training for nursing staff became a priority in many health care agencies (Lego, 1975). Neo-Freudian theories played a major role in the formation of 'developmental' nursing models. One may include in this category the work of Peplau (1952) and to a lesser extent Orlando (1961) and Travelbee (1966).

In the United Kingdom less emphasis was placed on the psychotherapeutic model. In 1962 the General Nursing Council for Scotland stressed that it was important for psychiatric nurses to take on a psychotherapeutic role (Cormack, 1981). However little training or practice was carried out to enable nurses to get the necessary skills. It came as a surprise therefore that in 1968 the Ministry of Health published a report maintaining that: "Some nurses have an active psychotherapeutic role an all carried out supportive psychotherapy to some degree." (Ministry of Health, 1968 p.6). This bore little resemblance to reality for, as Finch (1986) maintained, most psychiatric nurses did not practice psychotherapy in the strict sense of the word.

Research studies from both sides of the Atlantic show that psychiatric nurses can benefit from an understanding of the psychotherapeutic model (Lego, 1975; Altschul and Simpson, 1977). Denn (1975) found that those nurses who had a working knowledge of psychodynamics gave above average nursing care. Jones (1983) concluded that patients who had palpitations due to anxiety improved greatly when they were able to discuss their feelings with nurses who appreciated the psychological mechanisms involved. In the studies referenced, the researchers are not in agreement as to what constitutes psychotherapy and it is difficult to get consistency in definitions. Nevertheless in British literature there is concern that nurse psychotherapists are deserting their caring role (Martin, 1985). American research shows that this is not the case in the US (Lego, 1975). There is however opposition from another quarter, namely psychiatrists, some of whom do not like nurses to be involved in having an active treatment role with their patients.

It was reported in 1968 that psychiatrists rarely prescribed psychological treatment to be carried out by nursing staff (Ministry of Health, 1968). However Altschul (1972) found that some were more willing than others to allow nurses to practice psychotherapy. She discovered that much depended on the theoretical background of the doctor concerned. Psychiatrists who favoured the medical model or the sociotherapeutic model were prepared to permit nurses some psychotherapeutic function, whereas those who were psychotherapeutically oriented were less likely to condone nurse participation.

*The behavioural model*

The behavioural model has its origins in the learning theories of Pavlov (1927), Skinner (1938) and Bandura (1969). Although it does not ignore genetic or biological factors of aetiology, the behavioural frame of reference does view the medical model's quest for physical causes for mental disturbances as narrow and misleading. Hence it rejects the principle of mental disorder being an illness and concentrates on the alleviation of symptoms, which it believes to be the real problem for the patient (Clare, 1976).

The behavioural model is founded on the premise that all behaviour is learned and therefore can be unlearned. Mental illness is simply viewed as maladaptive behaviour that has been learned (Marks, 1986). Therefore using learning principles it follows that such maladaptive behaviour can be unlearned and replaced with more appropriate behaviour using techniques that produce behavioural change.

*Nursing's involvement with the behavioural model* As psychologists began to introduce behaviour changing techniques into psychiatric settings, some nurses, dismayed with the hierarchical ward structure, yearned for the autonomy inherent in the role of independent behavioural therapist. It was perceived by some as a means of leaving behind subservient custodialism and adopting a more active therapeutic role.

Psychologists soon became interested in carrying out operant conditioning techniques on long-stay psychiatric wards. However they realised that such an endeavour would require the co-operation of the nursing staff. In America, Ayllon and Michael (1959) introduced ward nurses to the principles of token economy. Altschul (1985) sees this as the earliest description of the nurse as a therapist. Ayllon and Michael (1959), pleased by the skill shown by the nursing staff, wrote a paper about the nurse as a 'behaviour engineer'. This paper inspired others to consider the nurses' role within the behavioural model. Marks, for instance, hypothesized that 'suitable psychiatric nurses' could be trained as behavioural therapists. He began his study in 1971 and by 1975 a national eighteen month course was endorsed by the Joint Board of Clinical Nursing Studies (Marks et al, 1977).

Research by Marks and others (1977) showed that nurses could use behavioural techniques successfully and get results equal to those of psychologists and psychiatrists with whom they were compared. It was found that nurse therapists could work independently, correctly assess patients and select appropriate treatment strategies. This study led Bird and his colleagues (1979) to conclude that the role of the nurse as therapist should be further developed.

Several research projects undertaken by Marks have produced interesting findings. In 1977 he concluded that behaviour therapy was the treatment of choice for 10% of all adult psychiatric out-patients. This figure increased to 12% in 1985 (Marks, 1985) and 13% in 1986 (Marks, 1986). Even considering that Marks may have an interest in the behavioural model, these figures still represented only one quarter of adults with neuroses - the 'tip of the psychiatric iceberg'.

As with the psychotherapeutic model, the behavioural model is a non-invasive framework whose goal is to involve the client in all aspects of therapy. In this regard the nurse therapist is an educator, teaching patients and their significant others to become active participants in the treatment process. Few mental health professionals will dispute the value of behaviour therapy for certain psychiatric disorders.

There is much anecdotal material concerning the impact of behavioural theory on psychiatric nursing. Although the empirical studies are few in number the investigators cited above were in agreement on a major point, that nurses functioning as behaviour therapists can be as therapeutically effective as psychologists and psychiatrists using the same methods.

However moral problems abound for nurses who attempt to put into practice the reward - punishment philosophy of operant conditioning. In many instances, cigarettes were the common currency for such rewards. But in some psychiatric hospitals where staff were inadequately prepared Ross (1981) reported a system where the necessities of life such as food and company were used as 'reinforcers'.

Barker and Fraser (1985) stated that the behavioural model, which was greeted with such enthusiasm in the 1960s, struggled to achieve anything like its true potential in the 1980s. The early belief that the mind was unimportant was rejected by many leading behaviourists. Bandura's social learning theory (1969) and Beck's cognitive theory (1976) encouraged the use of imagery, thought processes, memory and fantasy. In this regard the behavioural model moved a little towards the psychotherapeutic model.

## The sociotherapeutic model

The medical model, behavioural model and the psychotherapeutic model concentrate on individuals and aspects of their intrapersonal, interpersonal or intrapsychic functioning. The sociotherapeutic model adopts a broader focus and emphasizes not only the person but also the entire social environment in which they find themselves.

The sociotherapeutic model hypothesizes that mental disorder is a product of societal factors. These may incorporate overcrowding, noise, pollution (Siegal, 1980), competitiveness, poverty, stress (Clare, 1976), inadequate education and family instability (Caplan, 1964). Therefore the sociotherapeutic model shifts the cause of mental illness from the individual to society and social systems. Szasz (1961) maintained that society employs psychiatrists to incarcerate these 'so called nonconformists' in mental hospitals. If patients agreed to assimilate society's norms, they were discharged, if not, they were institutionalized.

The pernicious effects of institutionalization have been well documented (Jones, 1953; Barton, 1959; Wing and Brown, 1961). Goffman (1961) in his seminal work 'Asylums' showed how overcrowded, understaffed mental hospitals had used a "stripping process" and perpetuated the "us and them" syndrome.

It is possible that the paternalistic attitude seen among nurses who use the terms 'my patients' and 'my ward' helped to foster institutionalization. Thomas (1983) described nursing (in a misplaced effort to praise) as the glue that holds together hospitals as institutions. This was hardly surprising considering the custodial orientation of the nurse's role. But are nurses immune to the effects of institutionalization? This concern was expressed in the Rampton Report (DHSS, 1980) when it warned of the dangers of nurses succumbing to 'institutional inertia'.

*The therapeutic community* The therapeutic community became the vehicle by which the sociotherapeutic model was made manifest. Its basic philosophy arose from the model's emphasis on the following; an encouragement of personal relationships, an acceptance and tolerance of antisocial behaviour and  social interaction that generates the maturation and growth  of individual members of the community.

11

Cummings and Cummings (1962) identified the nurse as the keystone of the therapeutic community, a sentiment supported by many others (Altschul, 1962; Cohen and Strueing, 1965). In the literature the nurse was often called a Social engineer (Clare, 1976) or a sociotherapist (Hays, 1975).

Research by Rapoport (1960), a social anthropologist, identified four elements of the therapeutic community that were totally at odds with the medical model. These were: 'democratization', where patients and staff are jointly involved in decision making; 'permissiveness', where distressing behaviour is accepted and discussed; 'reality confrontation', where individual patients are confronted by the group for exhibiting unsocial behaviour; and 'communalism', where the hospital community functions as a therapeutic whole.

However several studies in the United States have highlighted problems with the therapeutic community. Visher and O'Sullivan (1970) found that staff were sceptical regarding the abilities of mental patients to organize and plan their own activities. Gardner and Gardner (1971) showed that sometimes 'democratization' worked so well that staff had difficulty influencing therapy or planning patient discharge.

Other research found that patients suffering from schizophrenia improved least on wards where patient responsibility was emphasized (Ellsworth et al, 1971). Within this aura of 'permissiveness', Bouras et al (1982) noted that anxiety rather than being contained was amplified resulting in apparent disorder. It is not surprising therefore that there are few true examples of therapeutic communities in the 1990s.

*Community care* When the ideology that underpinned the therapeutic community began to lose support in the 1980s the movement toward community care in the wider sense gained momentum. As a result the boundary line that served to define the limits of mental health care was extending. The new philosophy was given endorsement in the United Kingdom by a series of research reports. In the Worthing experiment of 1958, admissions had decreased by 59% in districts covered by a pilot community nurse scheme, whereas admissions rose by 4% in districts not covered by such a scheme (Sumner, 1981). Other studies supported these findings (Corrigan and Soni, 1977).

Community psychiatric nurses (C.P.N.) have emerged as a key group of professionals concerned with supporting the mentally ill in the community. Paykel et al (1982), in a prospective randomized controlled clinical trial, showed how C.P.N.s maintained patient improvement at the same level as psychiatrists. It was also noted in the same report that C.P.N.s exceeded psychiatrists in the giving of warmth and in achieving higher patient satisfaction.

The enthusiasm for psychiatric community care in the 1960s was accompanied by a critical reappraisal of this movement in the 1970s and 1980s. Without proper resources and organization it appears uncertain to some researchers whether community placement is the best type of care for people with mental disorders (Corrigan and Soni, 1977; Brooker, 1986). However recent research by White (1991) shows that a panel of psychiatric nurse experts were positive in their views about community care.

*The eclectic approach*

The conceptual frameworks outlined above show the richness and variety that pervade the field of psychiatric thought. Over the years some psychiatric nurses were open to changing their philosophical viewpoint. As a result nurses have functioned in the roles of doctors' assistants, individual psychotherapists, behaviour therapists and sociotherapists. Perhaps because of this variety of theoretical influences psychiatric nurses have been seen to adopt essentially an eclectic stance. In Britain Altschul (1980) recommended that in the complex field of psychiatry, no one model is always appropriate and nurses should use skills based on whatever approach they regard as helpful to a particular situation. Correspondingly, Reed (1987) argues that when caring for a patient with mental health problems American nurses tend to use information from all the available theories.

Clare (1976) recognized certain dangers with the eclectic approach. He believed that it is the soft option of "...a wishy-washy gutless mind that lacks decisiveness and clarity." (p.64). In this regard he was echoing the views of Eysenck (1971) who criticized those who subscribed to a 'mish-mash' of theories.

However there may be good reasons for adopting an eclectic stance. To survive in a continually changing world, psychiatric nursing should be open to modification and improvement. The use of one static model would be prescriptive, narrow and counter to the philosophy of holistic caregiving. Furthermore, models may be a product of their social context and some former thinking, becoming inappropriate over time.

Most practice professions have multiple models that make up what may be referred to as their 'theoretical toolkit'. Some practising psychiatric nurses have used non nursing models as the tools of their trade, selecting the one that they believe best suits a particular patient care situation. But apart from the medical model nurses have received little education or support in the use of these tools.

However, commenting on the use of non nursing models in psychiatric care, Barker (1991) states:

The continued influence of traditional viewpoints expressed through biological, psychodynamic and behavioural models are unhelpful. These models were more concerned with control than understanding. They emphasize repair work. (p.38).

Earlier Reed (1987) had argued that while non-nursing models provide valuable knowledge for practitioners, they may be incongruent with or limit nursing's perspective of significant care issues. Accordingly, she suggests that psychiatric nurses should not align their allegiance to any of the models reviewed above, but strive to use models of nursing that will show benefits not only for the patient but also for the profession. She concludes that only nursing models offer a means of clarifying mental nursing's conceptual base.

# 3 Literature review: nursing models

## Models for nursing or models of nursing?

Nurse academics throughout the world have currently formulated over forty nursing models. Of these twelve are British, while nearly all the rest have emanated from the North American continent. Most of these frameworks were not developed by psychiatric nurses. However, psychiatric nursing does not suffer from a paucity of theoretical approaches, as thirteen of the major nursing models have their basis in or are strongly connected with, mental health care. Barber (1986) argued that: "Many of those nursing models currently in vogue evolve from humanistic sources more akin to psychiatry than to general medicine or surgery..." (p.140).

*Clarification of terms*

There exists much semantic confusion in the nursing literature regarding the following terms: theory; conceptual model; conceptual theory; conceptual framework; theoretical framework; and paradigm. These terms seem to be used interchangeably and indiscriminately, hence causing confusion (Griffiths and Christenson, 1982), misunderstanding (Aggleton and Chalmers, 1986) and horror (Jackson, 1986) among practising nurses.

But practising nurses may not be alone in their confusion. Peplau referred to her work as: "...a set of concepts, a framework that can be applied to various kinds of nursing situations, but to call it a theory, I wouldn't." (cited in Suppe and Jacox, 1985 p243). Nevertheless, Stevens (1979) views Peplau's formulation as a theory, while Riehl and Roy (1980) call it a conceptual model. Similarly, Roy's work (1971) has been seen as a conceptual framework by Williams (1979), an ideology by Beckstrand (1980), a grand theory by Kim (1983) and as neither a model nor a theory by Webb (1986).

Orem's work (1958) has also been the object of some semantic ambiguity. The Nursing Theories Conference Group (1975) believe Orem has constructed a conceptual model, Johnson (1983) prefers to view it as a descriptive theory, Suppe and Jacox (1985) call it a conceptual framework and Rosenbaum (1986) favours the title macro-theory.

Despite these contrary opinions, it is widely believed in the literature that models lead to the identification of concepts and assumptions that when tested by research, will lead to the formation of theory (Fawcett, 1989). Models are therefore more abstract than theories. They present a generalized broader view of the phenomena under study, while nursing theories on the other hand, are more specific and precise, containing more clearly defined concepts with a narrower focus. Nonetheless an agreed upon definition for a nursing model is a major omission in the literature.

For this study the conceptualizations put forward by the major nurse theorists will be regarded as 'conceptual models'. This designation will be synonymous with the terms 'conceptual framework', 'nursing model' and 'model' and may be defined as:

> A mental or diagrammatic representation of nursing that is systematically constructed and assists nurses in organising their thinking about nursing and in the transfer of their thinking into practice for the benefit of the patient and the profession. (McKenna, 1989 p.762).

*The evolution of nursing models*

Although Florence Nightingale believed that the very elements of nursing were all but unknown, she expressed the firm belief that nursing knowledge should be distinct from medical knowledge (Nightingale, 1859, 1980). Having identified the individual - environment relationship as a prerequisite for health she is credited with laying the foundations for the development of nursing as a science.

At the turn of the century, Nightingale's early efforts were eclipsed by the adoption of the medical model that was to permeate nurse education and practice. The resultant theoretical hiatus in nursing persisted until the mid twentieth century. The following reasons have been put forward to explain why renewed attempts at conceptualizing nursing should have occurred in the 1950s:

1    The need to develop a scientific basis for nursing (Wald and Leonard, 1964);
2    The quest for professional status (Murphy, 1971);
3    Disenchantment with the medical model (Jacox, 1974);
4    The arrival of university education for nurses (Altschul, 1978);

5    The increased expectations and involvement of the patient (Ellis, 1982).

Mental health nursing took the lead in the reappearance of theoretical thinking among nurses. Peplau, a psychiatric nurse, is credited with formulating the first contemporary conceptual framework for nursing. Her work (Peplau, 1952) not only influenced, but formed the basis for, later attempts to develop nursing models. Henderson (1955), Orem (1958), Johnson (1959) and Hall (1959) followed Peplau's lead by focusing upon the importance of interpersonal relations. Their work was largely concerned with concept identification and nurse historians refer to these pioneers as the 'conceptualists' (Meleis, 1985).

The 1960s saw the publication of conceptual frameworks by Abdellah (1960), Orlando (1961), Wiedenbach (1964), Levine (1966), Travelbee (1966) and King (1968). Of these formulations Abdellah, Orlando and Travelbee were undoubtedly influenced by Peplau, with the latter two theorists concentrating particularly on psychiatric nursing.

The rapid growth in the number of nursing models witnessed in the 1960s continued into the 1970s with the introduction of models by Roy (1970), Rogers (1970), Neuman (1972), Riehl (1974), Adam (1975), Patterson and Zderad (1976), Leininger (1978), Watson (1979) and Newman (1979). Of these theorists, Neuman, Patterson, Leininger, Watson and Riehl have all specialized and worked extensively in psychiatric nursing.

Although the 1980s were characterized by an acceptance of the significance of nursing models, in America at least there was a slowing down in the number of nursing models being formulated. Established theorists began revising their work and examining how the status of theory might be achieved, while Parse (1981) and Fitzpatrick (1983) built their ideas on the work of another nurse theorist, namely Rogers (1970). This represented a new and interesting departure in the development of nursing models.

The evolution of nursing models between the 1950s and the 1970s was characterized by an adherence to logical positivism where the hypothetico-deductive view of science was preferred (Whall, 1989). In the late 1970s and 1980's the phenomenological approach came into favour reflected in the more humanistic models of Patterson and Zderad (1976), Newman (1979), Parse (1981) and Fitzpatrick (1983). This shift in theoretical approach coincides with the increased appearance of qualitative methods within nursing research a fact not unnoticed by Field and Morse (1985).

The major influence of psychiatric nursing on the early development of nursing models appears to have diminished in the 1970s. The reasons for this are unclear. Dumas (1978), noted this decline and urged psychiatric nurses to turn their attention once more to the development of relevant conceptual frameworks for mental health care.

Although Florence Nightingale identified her nursing concepts in nineteenth century England, the United Kingdom does not boast a tradition of nursing model development. However, Greaves (1984) believes that a look at the English nursing scene today is a view of the American nursing scene of yesterday. As if to reflect this, in the last decade several nurses have formulated conceptual models in Britain. Among these are Roper et al (1980), McFarlane (1982), Stockwell (1985), Wright (1986), Castledine (1986), Clark (1986), Minshull et al (1986), Green (1988), Bogdanovic (1989), Friend (1990) and Yoo (1991). Although Clark (1986) claims that her model is suitable for psychiatric nursing and Roper's model has been used extensively in this field, Stockwell's 'Enhancement' model is the only one designed specifically with the psychiatric patient in mind.

When considering the use of nursing models, it is important to examine the social context that accompanied their introduction into British psychiatric nursing in the first place. In the late 1970s and 1980s nursing was undergoing tremendous social change. The move from a traditional task-centred activity to a more patient-focused problem solving approach was a vitally important step for nursing at that time. There was also an increase in the number of graduate and post graduate nursing degrees courses at tertiary education establishments. This had the effect of stimulating an in-depth analysis concerning the appropriateness of non-nursing models. The lack of impact made by the psychotherapeutic model was noted and the narrow focus of the behavioural model was examined and found wanting (Barker, 1990).

Further, the patriarchal authority over women and womens' work symbolized by the medical model was recognized as having no place in modern nursing (Barker, 1990). Nurses wished to reject the handmaiden image and be recognized by society as professionals in their own right. However, while trying to escape from subservience to the psychiatrist there was the fear that the adoption of psychological models would lead nurse therapists to be little more than psychologists' assistants (Wilson-Barnett, 1976).

In addition, the emergence of new mental health legislation helped in altering the nurses' perception of patients. No longer was it legitimate to view them as passive hosts of a disease process; they became an active holistic individual. Quality assurance programmes were being introduced with an emphasis on consumerism and individuals were being given more rights culminating in the Patients' Charters

(DHSS, 1992). Psychiatric nurses were also beginning to view care as their central concern rather than looking to the medical model of cure for professional validation. Many believed that patient-centred nursing models were vehicles for actualising these new philosophies (Reed, 1987).

*Research on nursing models*

Historically, scant attention has been paid to the empirical study of nursing models and research into their use in mental health care is conspicuous by its scarcity. This is disturbing considering the widespread application of them into education and practice. In a recent British book Fraser (1990) admitted that for many nursing models "there is not a great deal of research available to date." (p.3). Therefore one must look to the United States for most of the investigations in this field.

Silva (1986) found sixty two empirical studies that used nursing models as frameworks to underpin their research. However these studies were aimed at testing theory; they were not concerned with the selection of, use of or attitudes towards nursing models. Tables 3.1 and 3.2 show that exploratory studies of this latter type are few.

One of the first descriptive studies on models of nursing was undertaken by Hall (1979). The researcher's report of her study is remarkably brief and methodological issues such as questionnaire psychometrics are not discussed. In fact only a few of the studies outlined in Tables 3.1 and 3.2 included any in depth discussion on the research methods used.

Hagemeier and Hunt (1979) found that most of their student nurse respondents had a positive image of nursing models. The researchers conclude that the students' use of a nursing model during training positively influences their professional practice later. However the study was limited to 69 respondents from the same school of nursing and the questionnaire was composed of only 13 items.

In Canada, Martin and Kirkpatrick (1987) undertook a survey on models as they apply to psychiatric nursing. Although most of the 64 respondents were familiar with Peplau's model only 34% used it in practice. Regarding how well prepared respondents believed they were to explain the model with which they were familiar, only 5% felt they were 'extremely well prepared'.

19

**Table 3.1. Descriptive research from North America on nursing models**

| RESEARCH | YEAR | UNITS OF STUDY | AIM OF STUDY | INSTRUMENTS | FINDINGS |
|---|---|---|---|---|---|
| Hall | 1979 | 144 nursing schools offering baccalaureate master's and doctoral programmes. | Which models are used for curricula and trends in the use of models? | Five part postal questionnaire. | Baccaleauteate programmes used models more than other programmes. Mostly used Roy, Orem, Rogers, Levine, Johnson and King. |
| Hagmiere & Hunt | 1979 | 150 graduates (69 responded) | Are teaching strategies effective and are the graduates using models in their practice? | Thirteen item likert-type questionnaire. | 53% positive view of models, most had understood models. 63% found them useful, 29% undecided. |
| Martin & Kirkpatrick | 1987 | 107 mental health nurses in Canada. (60% response rate). | Which models are staff familiar with, and do they use them? | Self report practice questionnaire | 22% always used a model, 5% never, 29% sometimes. 85% were familiar with Peplau. |
| Jacobson | 1987 | Master and doctoral students and their faculty staff. (691 respondents). | Which models are respondents familiar with, do they use them and how do they view them? | Forty three item questionnaire. | Familiar with Orem, Rogers, Peplau, King, Neuman, Johnson, Peplau and Levine. 35% use models. 76% are enthusiastic. |
| Salanders & Dietz-Omar | 1991 | Nurses prior to, during and after a course on nursing theory. | Do models help nurses with clinical decision making? | ? | Model do provide a frame of reference for clinical decision making. |

**Table 3.2. Descriptive research from Great Britain and Ireland on nursing models**

| RESEARCH | YEAR | UNITS OF STUDY | AIM OF STUDY | INSTRUMENTS | FINDINGS |
|---|---|---|---|---|---|
| Chavasse | 1987 | Application of nursing models with two patients | What effect does the application of three nursing models have? (Roy, Roper et al and Orem)? | Case study approach. | Roper et al's model inadequate for younger patients. Very few nurses could understand Roy's model. |
| Jukes | 1988 | Senior nurses and senior tutors in ten English Health Authorities. | Which assessment models are used in mental handicap and how important are models for such care? | Postal questionnaire. | Nursing models are mostly unused and tend to be for classroom application only. |
| Midgely | 1988 | 135 midwifery training schools. | Do midwifery schools use nursing models and if so, which ones? | Postal questionnaire. | Seventy schools did not use a nursing model, twenty four did; those that did - used Orem's model. |
| Mason and Chanley | 1990 | Forty primary nurses in ten special hospitals. | What model do respondents use and are they effective? | Semi-structured inter-view schedule. | Orem's model was used on five wards, Roper, Henderson and Riehl's models on two wards, Roy's model on three wards and Roger's model on one ward. 80% felt models were not effective, 15% felt they were. |

Jacobson (1987) in his study found that faculty members were more enthusiastic about models than their students. In the main it appears to be a well planned and executed survey. However, bias in the selection of potential respondents may have occurred because 'contact persons' in the target schools were relied upon to supply the names of eligible respondents.

In Salanders and Dietz-Omar's study (1991) data were collected from nurses at three points in time: prior to a nursing theory course, at the completion of the course and two years following completion of the course. At the first data collection point respondents were neutral in their responses. However at the two latter data collection points the respondents believed that nursing models did provide a frame of reference for clinical decision making in their practice.

Table 3.2 illustrates the main investigations into nursing models on this side of the Atlantic. They tend to be on a much smaller scale than the American studies. In Ireland, Chavasse (1987) used a case study approach to apply Roper et al, Roy and Orem's models to the care of two patients. She concluded that Roper et al's model was "adequate" for an elderly patient but "inadequate" for a younger patient. She also maintained that very few nurses "trained using the present nursing syllabus" could begin to understand Roy's model and parts of Orem's model are "fairly obscure".

In England Jukes (1988) found that Roper et al's model was favoured by senior nurse tutors in four out of the ten Health Authorities he surveyed. Henderson' model was favoured by two, Peplau's by one, Orem's by one and Roy's by one. Jukes does not mention how the respondents were selected. One must also question if senior tutors would necessarily be 'au fait' with current assessment strategies at patient care level.

Also in England, Midgley (1988) undertook research into the use of nursing models in midwifery. Responses from 135 midwifery training schools indicated that seventy of these schools did not use a model of nursing or the nursing process at all. Twenty four did use a nursing model and forty one used the nursing process only. Of those using a model most used Orem, 'some loosely' and some in combination with others.

A more recent English study by Mason and Chanley (1990) found that Orem's model was used more often than any other nursing model. Most of the respondents believed that nursing models were not effective. None of the fifteen percent who thought they were effective could produce evidence of effectiveness. Unfortunately the researchers give little or no details on how the respondents were selected nor on the research instrument.

To summarize the research in this field it can be seen that published investigations are few in number and generally tied to a self-report methodology. Most of the studies encountered in the literature were undertaken in nurse education and tend to concentrate on the report of findings rather than of method. This leaves the reader at a disadvantage if one is interested in replicating the studies or in generalising the findings to other areas. Studies from Britain and Ireland show that Roper et al's work appears to be the model of choice for education and practice whereas in the North American studies it is Orem's model that is most often used. Martin and Kirkpatrick's Canadian study is the exception where Peplau was the most frequently used model. Most of these studies were limited by size and methodological rigour. Therefore in the absence of follow up research they contribute insufficiently to current knowledge on how nursing models are selected or on how practitioners view nursing models.

*Theoretical classification of nursing models*

Regardless of discipline all models have their roots in a theory or group of theories (Sorensen and Luckmann, 1986). Nursing models are no exception. Their theoretical foundations have been identified as 'systems' theory, 'interactional' theory and 'developmental' theory (Riehl and Roy, 1974). Some models also have a large behavioural component (McClymont, 1985) and hence the 'behavioural' theory is sometimes included as an additional theoretical category (Chapman, 1985).

However these classifications are not exclusive in their emphasis and assignment to each category may be arbitrary. This has led to disagreement among nurses as to what theoretical grouping a particular model belongs. For instance, Orem's work has been seen as: a System's model by Suppe and Jacox (1985); an Interactional model by Greaves (1984); a Developmental model by McFarlane (1986); and a Behavioural model by Chapman (1985). Nevertheless this method of categorization has been considered a valid manner of classifying nursing models (Thibodeau, 1983).

*Systems models* These nursing models are largely based upon the General Systems theory as put forward by Von Bertlanffy (1951). A 'system' is simply a collection of parts that interrelate as a whole entity for a particular purpose. If the system can affect and in turn be affected by, outside influences it is called an 'open system'. The work of Johnson (1959), Roy (1970), Neuman (1972), Parse (1981) and Fitzpatrick (1983) are examples of 'systems models'.

*Interactional models* Interactional models are seen as having their basis in Symbolic Interactionist theory (Blumer, 1969). This theory emphasizes the relationships between people and the roles they play in society. Nursing is seen as a social activity, an interactional process between the nurse and the patient. It requires the nurse to empathize with patients to understand how they see their present state of wellness or illness. Among the better known 'interactional models' are: Orlando (1961); Levine (1966); King (1968); Riehl (1974); and Patterson and Zderad (1976).

*Developmental models*  Developmental models take their origins from the work of Freud (1949) and Sullivan (1953). The central themes are growth, development, maturation and change. Within developmental theory it is argued that from the moment of conception to the moment of death, human beings are constantly developing. This maturation may be social, physiological, psychological or spiritual. Development is seen as an ongoing process in which individuals must pass through various stages and with each transition they achieve greater self responsibility. Nursing involves removing or preventing barriers to this natural developmental process. One may include among the 'developmental models' the work of Peplau (1952), Travelbee (1964) and Newman (1979).

*Behavioural models*  These conceptual frameworks owe much to the theoretical formulations of Abraham Maslow (1954). Because of this, they are often called 'human needs models' (Meleis, 1985). Behavioural models assume that individuals normally function in society by their own efforts, that is, they meet their needs, carry out their activities of living and undertake their self care requirements. Therefore independence in basic human needs is the focus for nursing action within 'behavioural models'. This category includes the work of Henderson (1955), Orem (1958), Wiedenbach (1964), Rogers (1970), Roper et al (1980) and Minshull et al (1986).

Philosophically two main methods for the development of theory have been identified: the inductive approach and the deductive approach (Harre, 1972). The inductive method leads to the development of theory based upon evidence drawn from observation and personal experience. In this case the 'theorist' is reasoning from the 'specific' to the 'general'. In contrast the deductive method leads to the development of theory from existing theories where reasoning is from the 'general' to the 'specific'. Although some nursing theorists maintain that they derived their models from observing practice (Roy, 1971; Orem, 1980), most take as their starting point one or more of those theoretical bases outlined above. Therefore it could be argued that if nursing models are deduced from the existing theories of other disciplines they may have difficulty explaining the actuality of nursing practice. This failure of models to reflect reality and the implications this has for the 'real-ideal gap' will be expanded upon in part two of this study.

*The essential elements of nursing models*

Regardless of how nursing models are categorized, there is agreement that each one must include views on certain central concepts. In 1974 Torres and Yura surveyed a sample of 50 American baccalaureate nursing programmes accredited by the National League of Nursing. They concluded that the elements of Nursing, health, man and society were central to all the programmes reviewed. These concepts have more recently been refined as; Nursing, Health, the Person and the Environment. When referring to these elements Fawcett (1984) uses the term 'metaparadigm', while Meleis (1985) calls them 'domain concepts'. Fawcett (1989) defined a 'metaparadigm' as "The global perspective of any discipline  that acts as an encapsulating structure within which conceptual frameworks develop." (p.67). Most professions have a single metaparadigm from which many models emerge, - contemporary nursing appears to have reached this level of theoretical development.

During the 1970s and 1980s nursing authors wrote extensively about the importance of these major elements for nursing science. The argument has been put forward that unless a conceptual framework includes assumptions about Nursing, Health, Person and Environment it cannot be considered a nursing model (Fitzpatrick and Whall, 1989).

According to Fitzpatrick et al (1982) these four elements have a particular significance for the psychiatric nurse. Smith (1986) believes that if nursing models are to be employed in psychiatry these concepts must be explicated. Reed (1987), while developing a model for psychiatric nursing practice, stresses the interdependence of these concepts. She discusses the fluidity and interconnections that must exist between them if psychiatric nursing is to develop a unique body of knowledge.

Although each nursing model deals with the four essential elements of the metaparadigm, they may stress different aspects and see them in different relations to one another (See Figure 3.1). Therefore how nursing, health, person and environment are described and defined vary greatly from theorist to theorist. According to Chong Choi (1986), such a diversity of assumptions concerning the same concepts will only serve to enrich nursing as a profession.

**Figure 3.1. The relationship between the metaparadigm and nursing models (Adapted from  Fawcett, 1989)**

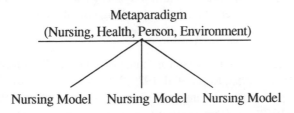

Metaparadigm
(Nursing, Health, Person, Environment)

Nursing Model     Nursing Model     Nursing Model

The complete metaparadigm has its dissenters. For example, Stevens (1979) excludes Environment, while Kim (1983) excludes Health. Others believe that Nursing should be omitted as an element, maintaining that its inclusion is a redundancy in terms (Rosenbaum, 1986). However since most authors support the metaparadigm in its entirety an overview of how different theorists deal with the four elements will show the similarities and differences in their thinking.

*Health* Within nursing models, health has been represented as a level of adaptation (Levine, 1966; King, 1968; Roy, 1970), an appropriate level of independence (Peplau, 1952; Roper et al, 1980; Minshull et al, 1986), a state of wholeness (Rogers, 1970; Riehl, 1974; Orem, 1980) or a desired value (Johnson, 1959; Travelbee, 1966). Neuman (1972) and Patterson and Zderad (1976) discuss health as 'wellness', while Orlando (1961) outlines the importance of 'mental and physical comfort'.

*Nursing* Among nursing academics, there is still no generally accepted definition of 'nursing'. This may be because, as Wetherston (1979) noted, we are dealing with a complex phenomenon. Such complexity is reflected in how nursing is explicated within conceptual frameworks.

Some nursing models view 'nursing' as, 'assisting as necessary' (Orem, 1958; Roper et al, 1980; Minshull et al, 1986). Those frameworks that have their focus on psychiatric care tend to envisage 'nursing' as 'an interpersonal process' (Peplau, 1952; Orlando, 1961; Travelbee, 1966). King (1968) and Riehl (1974), firm advocates of interactional theory, believe nursing is about 'social interaction'.

Other descriptions of nursing include, 'supporting the patients' adaptation' (Levine, 1966; Roy, 1970; Rogers, 1970), 'helping patient achieve equilibrium' (Johnson, 1959) 'participating with the patient's health experiences' (Parse, 1981), 'enhancing the developmental process towards health' (Fitzpatrick, 1983), 'assisting persons to utilize their own resources' (Newman, 1979) and 'intervening at primary, secondary and tertiary levels of prevention (Neuman, 1972).

*Person* Over the years nursing's view of the person has changed from being an anatomical and physiological entity with mind-body dichotomy, to being an individual with biological, spiritual, emotional, social and cognitive dimensions. This 'holistic' image tends to permeate most nursing models.

Many nurse theorists see the person as 'someone who has differing and changing needs' (Henderson, 1955; Roper et al, 1980; Minshull et al, 1986). Orem (1971) focuses on the person as a self care agent. Parse (1981), Fitzpatrick (1983), Neuman (1972), King (1968) and Johnson (1958) see the person as an 'open system', while

Rogers (1970) and Newman (1979) describe him/her as an 'energy field'.

Several other descriptions exist. For example an 'adapter to stress' (Levine, 1966; Roy, 1970), a 'behaving human organism' (Orlando, 1961), an 'incarnate being' (Patterson and Zderad, 1976), an 'evolving irreplaceable individual' (Travelbee, 1966) or simply 'one who has intrinsic value' (Riehl, 1974).

*Environment*  Nurse theorists tend to view the environment as not just what is external to the person, but many also recognize an 'internal environment' (Roy, 1970; Orem, 1980; Neuman, 1972). Other models portray the environment as the 'arena where the person functions', 'where he gets his sustenance' and 'where threats to his integrity arise' (Orlando, 1961; Travelbee, 1966;  Riehl, 1974).

Newman (1979) and Rogers (1970) consider the environment to be an 'energy field' that is part of the 'life process'. King (1968) and Fitzpatrick (1983), in keeping with their views on the 'person', believe the environment to be an 'open system' in interaction with human beings.  Corresponding with her assumptions regarding interpersonal relationships, Peplau (1952) describes the environment as 'microcosms of significant others with whom the person interacts'

Thus, it has been shown that, although all nursing models deal with health, nursing, person and environment, they tend to view them from different perspectives. There are, of course, some commonalities and one can see the influences of the underlying systems, interactional, developmental and behavioural theories. Nevertheless the basic metaparadigm elements have been moulded to suit the different perspectives of the individual theorists. Therefore each model is uniquely different.

*Selecting an  appropriate nursing model*

He that knows theory, but not practice, does not know   the whole theory.
(Perkins, 1965 p.34).

Since psychiatric assessment, planning, intervention and evaluation will differ depending on which conceptual framework is in use (Collister, 1986; Smith, 1986) it is important to make an appropriate choice. Although some authors maintain that most models are applicable to any setting (Riehl and Roy, 1974), the choice of one model for application throughout an area is seen as imprudent (Burgess and Lazare, 1973).  Stevens (1979) asks whether patients and nurses should have to put up with a model with a less desirable 'fit' for the sake of conformity.  There exists, therefore, a body of opinion which strongly stresses the need to employ different nursing models to suit different patient populations.

It is not uncommon for a nursing model to be imposed with little or no discussion with practitioners. Chapman (1990) relates a typical United Kingdom selection strategy:

> Senior nurses and tutors decide which model will be used in each ward or unit and charge nurses and staff are requested to become acquainted with it (with varying amounts of help from the school and service side) and to interpret and use it on their ward. Enthusiasm...may understandably be grudging, so the minimum is done to satisfy the requirements. (p.14).

*Issues for consideration when selecting an appropriate nursing model*

In her study Openshaw (1984) provides an excellent overview of how practising nurses make decisions. She examined several studies and theories on the subject and concluded that little is actually known about the complex processes involved in decision making.

Several factors, including intelligence, expectations, memory and information overload affect an individual's decision making ability. It is also possible that when faced with different options the decisions people make are influenced by how the options are presented. For instance, Tversky and Kahneman (1981) presented health care personnel with a decision task concerning two alternative immunization programmes against a lethal disease. They found that wording the problem from a statement of lives saved to one of lives lost produced differing results. Therefore, decisions made regarding the selection of a nursing model may be influenced by the language of different models and how they are presented to practising nurses. This issue will be developed further when parsimony and the suitability of American models are addressed below.

Vinokuv (1971) formulated models of decision making based upon the work of Lewin (1951). Vinokuv believed that in making a decision between two or more courses of action it is rational to seek the maximum benefit to oneself. When faced with alternatives the rational individual chooses the alternative with the most desirable outcomes. Therefore it is possible that when nurses are selecting a nursing model they will choose one that will suit them rather than the patients.

The literature highlights several other factors that may affect the selection of a nursing model.

*Practitioner's knowledge*   Chavasse (1987) believes that the level of nursing knowledge has a great influence on the appropriateness of the chosen model.

However, it may not be realistic to expect the busy practitioner to have knowledge of any more than a small number of conceptual frameworks. This has obvious implications for nurse education. Nurse teachers have to decide whether it is better for students to have a good understanding of a few nursing models or a superficial understanding of many.

*Merging and adapting conceptual frameworks* The idea that different concepts can be selected from several nursing models and applied in the clinical area as one framework is supported by some (Fawcett, 1980), but seen as totally untenable by others. Webb (1986b) argues that such a strategy would lead to loss of coherence and rigour, the introduction of contradiction and theoretical status being compromized.

*Ethical, social and political implications* All models have their strengths and limitations. Therefore by selecting a particular model a nurse is choosing not to look at certain factors while focusing on others. If nurses commit themselves to high standards in the promotion of adaptation, independence or self care, they will be held accountable by society for this service. Furthermore, one could ask, should nurses use force, however subtly, to make patients self caring? Webb (1986) believes that Orem's work (1980) is more suited to the private health insurance sector. If self care or dependant self care is encouraged in hospital the patient may get discharged earlier. This may lead to insurance companies having to pay smaller health care bills. However, if discharged too early, possible relapse and complications could be expensive. This would have workload implications for community staff.

*Intuition or scientific fact* Should the selection of a nursing model be based upon scientific enquiry or merely the 'gut reaction' of the nurse? Silva (1977) urged nurses to value truths arrived at by intuition and introspection as much as those arrived at by scientific experimentation, while Bishop (1986) stressed that selection must be made on more logical grounds. Considering the benefits of both strategies it would be wrong for nurses to be polarized on this issue.

*The use of multiple models* Although the selection within one hospital of different models for different patient groups may be a desirable and recommended stratagem, it may lead to great problems with inservice training and documentation. The luxury of such diversity may be expensive and complex. Those who would be 'crossing the lines' between different areas such as nursing officers, tutorial staff and paramedical staff would require a high degree of theoretical sophistication.

*Restrictiveness of models* In discussing the application of models to psychiatric nursing, Dienemann (1976) and Smith (1986) concluded that every model is limited by its own assumptions and therefore no one model will be able to deal with all eventualities. Smith (1986) states that many psychiatric nurses express incredulity and disbelief at the thought that psychiatric patients should be encouraged to undertake self care. Collister (1986) maintains that Orem's model (1980) or Henderson's model (1966) have proved difficult to use in psychiatric nursing as frameworks for assessment or for identifying patient care goals. Reed and Robbins (1991) question the validity of Roper et al's model (1980) in caring for patients. They argue that rather than contributing to nursing excellence its restrictiveness may undermine the confidence and competence of the skilled nurse. However if models are seen as 'tools' it may be more proper to blame the selector and user of the tool rather than the tool itself.

*Model complexity*   "The language of science cannot be freed from ambiguity any more than poetry can." (Bronowski, 1980 p.121). 'Occam's Razor' states that 'the simplest theory is to be selected from among all other theories that fit the facts as we know them' (Oxford Dictionary of Quotations, 1988 p.364). This traditional belief is synonymous with the modern idea of 'parsimony'. Parsimony dictates that a good model is stated in the most simple terms possible (George, 1985). Although acknowledging the over use of jargon in some nursing models, Ellis (1968) states that a model must have complexity to be significant. After all, since the concepts under study are abstract, precise theoretical parlance must, by necessity, be complex.

*The suitability of American models*   "Americanisms... are only for those who are Americans and nothing else." (Roosevelt, 1913 p.34). Most nursing models have their origin in the United States. A question has been posed whether these conceptual frameworks are transferable to nursing practice in Britain (Girot, 1990). Wright (1990) suggests that there is nothing wrong with nurses from different nations swapping ideas, but the application of one group's practices to the other may not always be appropriate. Most of the literature on this issue is anecdotal and so no definitive conclusion can be drawn. However, if British nurses continually look towards America for conceptual guidance, the imported models will have to be adapted to ensure their validity within the British health service.

*Staff attitudes*   Loughlin (1988) claims that there exists at clinical level a distrust of nursing models, a claim echoed by Smith (1986) who believes that in psychiatric nursing the abhorrence felt towards the nursing process has been transferred to nursing models. Hawkett (1989) argues that nurses view models with suspicion and describe them as 'woolly and impractical', while Lister (1987) believes "no particular model has gained popularity in psychiatric nursing." (p.42).

*Criteria for the selection of a nursing model*

*Type of patient*  When considering the choice of a model for psychiatric nursing practice it seems obvious that the main selection criterion should focus on what model is best for the patients and how it meets their needs. This emphasis has been supported by Walsh (1990) and Kershaw (1990).

*Health care setting*  This second criterion is related to the first but concentrates on contextual factors in the patient care setting. Clark (1982) likened nursing models to maps that guide our practice. To take this analogy a step further, we require a different map to suit the specific terrain in which we find ourselves. Collister (1986) emphasizes the importance of considering the 'care arena' when choosing an appropriate model for psychiatric nursing. According to George (1985) nurses from different units should select their own nursing model depending on the fit of that model to the function of that unit.

*Parsimony and simplicity*  Although the idea of parsimony has already been discussed it is very important as a criterion for selecting an appropriate practice model. Salvage (1985) asserts that a nursing model must be easily understood if it is to 'cut any ice' with the busy nurse and obviously nurses would have difficulty using a nursing model if they cannot understand it. In her study (see p.21) Chavasse (1987) concluded that very few Irish nurses trained within the 'current curriculum' would be able to understand Roy's (1970) and Orem's (1980) models. Similarly, Jackson (1986) wonders what use elaborate lines and circles are if nurses cannot use them to guide their practice.

*Logistics for the selection of a nursing model*

Adam (1980) outlined five possible ways to select a suitable model for nursing practice:

1.  A committee or group make their choice from existing models;
2.  Every concerned individual participates in a comparative study of several models;
3.  An entire group develops its own specific nursing model;
4.  A group chooses an existing model, but plans to develop their own;
5.  'Bits and pieces' are taken from several models to form an eclectic model. (p.82).

Adam points out that, although the second method may be a lengthy process, in the end the change will be more lasting if every concerned individual has been part of the decision making process. The theories of change from which this fundamental tenet is derived will be explored in greater detail in part two of this study. Suffice to state here that accepting a decision imposed by others often means a short lived allegiance.

*Theoretical bases as a method for model selection*    As discussed above, every nursing model has its roots in one or more of the following theories: systems theory; interactional theory; developmental theory; and behavioural theory. Aggleton and Chalmers (1986) believe that these broad theoretical foundations could help nurses make some preliminary decisions about the type of nursing model that is most appropriate to their patients. Maloney (1984) appears to be in full agreement with this belief, maintaining that psychiatric nurses exposing an interactional approach to human nature are unlikely to select a system model as their major theoretical position.

*Nurses' values and beliefs as a basis for choice*   "We all have a private image of nursing practice and in turn these images influence our interpretation of data, our decisions and our actions." (Reilly, 1975 p.567). It is generally supported in the literature that all nurses have a personal conception in their minds regarding the central components of their craft. This conception is believed to be based upon the individual nurse's values and beliefs concerning 'nursing', 'health', 'person' and 'environment' (Sorensen and Luckmann, 1986). These values and beliefs have been called the practitioner's own 'implicit nursing model' (Collister, 1988). Therefore a nurse's personal model contains ideas and assumptions about the metaparadigm (Fawcett, 1989).

McFarlane (1986) wrote:

> Most nurses have a rough picture of nursing that includes ideas about the nature and role of the patient and the nurse, the environment... in which nursing takes place and the major field of nursing function, i.e. health care and the nature of nursing methods or action. (p.3).

Although Jackson (1986) claims that most nurses are able to reveal these private images, in the reality of the practice situation they are seldom articulated. Hence they are mostly hidden in the nurse's mind rather than being made explicit. In a Canadian study, Field (1983) examined the implicit models of four nurses. Findings suggested that they guided the nurses' practice but, because of their unarticulated form, could not be shared with others. However if these implicit models cannot be shared they remain useful only to oneself. There is also the danger that because of this concealment, these 'personal guides to practice' may be incomplete, unproven, inconsistent and muddled.

32

Like the nurse's personal model, internationally recognized nursing frameworks are not 'value free'. They also were initially founded on the "private images" (Fawcett, 1980), "individual views" (Smith, 1986), "mental pictures" (Adam, 1980) and "rich insights" (Bohny, 1980), of their originators. As referred to elsewhere in this chapter, these 'images', 'views', 'pictures' and 'insights' also tend to concentrate on nursing, health, person and the environment and the relationships between these elements.

Field (1983) stresses that practising nurses must try to translate the 'know how' of practice into the 'know that' of models. In this way the 'theory practice gap' could be closed. Therefore, since every nurse has a personal model concerning how they view the metaparadigm components and recognized models also have this focus, it is possible that a nurse could select a framework that best reflects her beliefs and values related to these elements (Rogers, 1986). Collister (1988) sees this as an essential requisite if the model is to fit the reality of psychiatric care. When considering the selection of a model for psychiatric nursing it has been stated that: "Although it is advisable to practice what we preach, it is difficult, if not impossible to practice what we could not preach from the heart." (Mansfield, 1980 p.35).

The following steps are offered by Fawcett (1984) as a guide for the selection of an appropriate nursing model:

Her beliefs and values about the person, the environment, health and nursing will direct the nurse to look for a model congruent with these ideas. The nurse must then...compare the content of the model with her philosophic statements and select the conceptual model that most closely matches these philosophic beliefs. (p.48).

According to Adam (1980) and Webb (1986b) if nurses cannot accept how some concepts are treated within a particular nursing model they should reject that model and choose another whose concepts would be more compatible with their own. In this way congruence will be reached between the nurses' clinical orientation and a recognized conceptual framework. Adam (1985) feels that their final choice will indicate for these nurses what they have always believed about nursing but could not articulate in such a clear and distinct manner.

In their Canadian research, Martin and Kirkpatrick (1987) asked psychiatric nurse practitioners to identify whom they believe should select a nursing model for patient care. Results showed that 22% felt that nurse administrators should choose, 3.2% nominated the ward manager, 1% suggested nurse teachers and 52% indicated that those individual nurses directly looking after the patient should select the most appropriate model.

None of the respondents in Martin and Kirkpatrick's study mentioned whether they believed the patient should be involved in the selection process. This is strange considering the emphasis on the patient as a partner in care. Gould (1989) argues that when selecting a nursing model the beliefs and values of the most important person concerned, the recipient of care cannot be ignored. However to date there has been no research which has involved the patient in this process. Therefore the following question remains unanswered: if nursing models are viewed as confusing by many professionals would patients not find them more confusing? If the answer is in the affirmative it may not be realistic to expect equal partnership between nurse and patient in the selection of a nursing model.

Most authors agree with Martin and Kirkpatrick that 'practising nurses' should be involved in the selection process. Farmer (1986) and Pearson (1986) both recommend the clinical manager of a unit to decide upon the most relevant nursing model. This may indeed be a valid nomination considering that many British studies have identified the ward sister as possessing the most knowledge and influence regarding clinical work orientation and practical expertise (Alexander and Orton, 1988).

Therefore the literature suggests that ward managers should try to match the philosophy of their implicit nursing model, built up over the years, with the philosophy of a recognized model of nursing practice. This can be done by considering the theoretical underpinnings of each model (Aggleton and Chalmers, 1986) and by seeking compatibility between how the nurse and how the model view 'nursing', 'health', 'person' and the 'environment' (Fawcett, 1984).

# 4 Methodology

## Design and method

The main aim of the first part of this study is to find out which nursing model(s) will ward sisters/charge nurses in long-stay psychiatric care select as suitable for use with their patients. It is also intended to collect information on the possible reasons for their choice and their opinions of nursing models. For the purposes of this study the designation 'ward manager' will be used to denote ward sister and charge nurse.

### Research questions

A.  What nursing model (from a predetermined list of options) will the majority of ward managers on long-stay psychiatric areas select as suitable for implementation with their care group?
B.  What theoretical basis do ward managers favour for nursing practice on long-stay psychiatric wards?
C.  What are the opinions of ward managers on long-stay psychiatric wards in Northern Ireland on nursing models?
D.  Is there a relationship between choice of nursing model and the demographic profile of ward manager (age, sex, length of time in psychiatric nursing, length of time in long-stay wards, nursing qualifications, educational background)?
E.  Is there a relationship between choice of nursing model and positive and/or negative opinions towards nursing models?

### Operational definitions

*Nursing model* A mental and/or diagrammatic representation of nursing that is systematically constructed and which assists nurses in organising their thinking about nursing and in the transfer of their thinking into practice for the benefit of the patient and for the profession as a whole.

*Long-stay psychiatric patients* Those psychiatric patients who do not require the facilities of the admission wards and are not currently treated within those areas designated as psychogeriatric, but who have spent two or more years in continuous hospitalization.

*Ward managers (Delphi 'experts')* The nurse or nurses who have the designation ward sister/charge nurse and hold responsibility at ward level for the nursing care of long-stay patients within the psychiatric hospitals of Northern Ireland.

*Theoretical bases* The developmental, systems, interactional and/or behavioural theories on which most nursing models are based.

*Model statement* How each nursing model explicates the central elements: 'Nursing', 'Health', 'Person' and 'Environment'.

*Nursing model consensus* The model statement(s) that is/are most appropriate to the care of long-stay psychiatric patients, as identified by the majority of ward managers ( > 51% ) working within that setting.

*Theoretical levels of research enquiry*

Diers (1979) identified four levels of research investigation based on the work of Dickoff and James (1968): factor searching studies, relation searching studies, association testing studies and causal-hypotheses testing studies.

The first part of this study represents a 'relation searching' study with aspects of a 'factor searching' study incorporated within it. This is an acceptable mixture (Diers, 1979 p.135). It represents the 'context of discovery' because it is an area that no one has investigated in depth before. Besides this, the aim is to describe and explore judgments, opinions and values and therefore the lack of available scientific data precludes hypothesis testing.

The elements of interest (nursing models, long-stay psychiatry, ward managers) have already been recognized and widely discussed in the literature, albeit in an unconnected fashion. Therefore these factors are known to exist, an important prerequisite of relation searching studies. Diers (1979) maintains that relation searching studies may be legitimately concerned with the relationship between a particular group of patients and their nursing needs. The current research project

36

focuses on the identification of a nursing model that respondents believe is most appropriate to the needs of long-stay psychiatric patients. It is also proposed to uncover any relationship between the respondents' choice of nursing model and their demographic profile or opinions towards nursing models.

## Selecting the research method

*The survey approach* If it is believed that answers to the research questions 'do exist at present' but must be sought in a systematic manner, Fox (1982) suggests that the survey approach be adopted. According to Phillips (1986), descriptive/exploratory surveys are aimed at identifying opinions, judgments, attitudes, values and relationships. Considering the level of enquiry, the research context, the research respondents and the lack of previous research in the area, a descriptive/exploratory survey design was considered the best approach.

Within the survey approach two main methods are available. These are observing and questioning. Previous British research on the psychiatric nurse has primarily used the observation method (Altschul, 1972; Towell, 1975; Cormack, 1976). However this method is mainly concerned with observing behaviour or environmental characteristics (Polit and Hungler, 1987) and is therefore, unsuitable to the phenomena under consideration in the first part of the present study.

Questioning is used to collect data on things that are not easily observable such as opinions and perceptions (Diers, 1979). In a survey that involves questioning, there is some spoken or written interaction between the researcher and the data source. This is a method unique to the social disciplines to which nursing belongs. In the present study the investigator believes that the answers to the research questions can best be obtained by asking the relevant respondents pertinent questions in a systematic scientific manner.

Within the questioning method, available data gathering techniques include the interview, the postal questionnaire, the critical incident technique, the repertory grid technique and the Delphi technique. To answer the main question posed the most suitable research exercise regarding time and costs (Reid, 1988), is the Delphi technique.

## The Delphi technique

I have brought golden opinions from all sorts of people. (Macbeth, vii p.31).

According to Dalkey and Helmer (1963) the Delphi technique may be defined as:

A method used to obtain the most reliable consensus of opinion of a group of experts by a series of intensive questionnaires interspersed with controlled feedback. (p.103).

With increasing usage, broader definitions have been put forward. For instance, Reid (1988) believes the 'Delphi' to be:

A method for the systematic collection and aggregation of informed judgment from a group of experts on specific questions and issues. (p.78).

The Delphi approach involves the presentation of a questionnaire or interview schedule to a panel of 'informed individuals' in a specific field of application to seek their opinion or judgment on a particular issue. After they have responded, the data are summarized and a new questionnaire is designed based solely on the results obtained from the first application. This second instrument is returned to each respondent and they are asked, in the light of the first round's results, to reconsider their initial judgment and to again return their responses to the researcher. Repeat rounds of this process may be carried out until agreement or a point of diminishing returns, has been reached.

In essence therefore the Delphi technique is a multistage approach with each stage building on the results of the previous one. Hitch and Murgatroyd (1983) see it resembling a meeting of experts, closely controlled by a chairperson who is adept at summing up the feelings of the meeting by reflecting the participants' own views back to them so that they can proceed further; the only difference is that the individual responses of the members are unknown to the others.

There is substantial evidence in the literature that in the first round of any Delphi investigation a wide divergence of individual opinion is typical. Nonetheless, after several iterations there is a tendency for respondents to converge towards consensus. Dalkey and Helmer (1963) saw this as almost inevitable considering the use of the feedback-response loop. An important issue among researchers planning to use the Delphi technique is an understanding of what is meant by 'consensus'. It has been posited that this should be equated with 51% agreement among respondents (Loughlin and Moore, 1979). It is difficult to find other authors who are as explicit as this.

*Reasons for choosing the Delphi technique* Linstone and Turoff (1975), who have edited the seminal work on 'Delphi', outline the following reasons why a researcher may choose this approach. The same justifications can reasonably apply to the present study:

1. The research problem does not lend itself to precise analytical techniques but can benefit from subjective judgments on a collective basis;
2. The research population may present diverse backgrounds concerning experience or expertise;
3. More subjects are needed than can effectively interact in a face to face exchange;
4. Time, cost and logistics would make frequent meeting of all the subjects unfeasible.

Farrell and Scherer (1983) maintain that the Delphi technique is suitable for areas where there are a lack of empirical data. This is presently the case concerning what nursing models would be most appropriate for psychiatric care. The 'Delphi' was seen as the correct procedure for structuring the responses of the subjects into a decision making process for the benefit of answering the research questions.

Reid (1988) emphasizes that the decision by any researcher to use the Delphi method centres around the available alternatives. The aim of this study was to help ward managers identify a suitable nursing model befitting the requirements of their particular care group. Used alone, the postal questionnaire or the interview schedule would undoubtedly give the investigator a wide range of opinions and judgments on various nursing models. However none of the alternative methods attempt to obtain information and consensus. Therefore the main advantage of the 'Delphi' for the present study is the achievement of agreement in a given area where none previously existed.

*The use of the Delphi technique in nursing research* Despite its existence as a survey approach since 1948 with over a thousand published utilizations (Linstone and Turoff, 1975), nurse researchers have been slow to adopt the Delphi technique as a suitable research method. This is beginning to change. Contemporary nursing literature shows increasing evidence of its use in a wide range of problem areas including nurse education, research priorities and the setting of standards.

In Canada in 1974, Bramwell and Hykawy used the Delphi approach to predict future occurrences in the realm of nurse education. The expertise required was elicited from thirteen nurse teachers over a four round application. More recently their compatriot, Limieux-Charles (1980) undertook a similar study to establish a 'blueprint' for nurse training in Ontario. In Northern Ireland, Reid (1985) set up a Delphi panel of nurse tutors to help in the identification and weighting of items for various practical nursing procedures.

Lindeman (1975), Oberst (1978) and Ventura and Waligora-Serafin (1981) in the United States and Bond and Bond (1982), Goodman (1986) and MacMillan (1989) in Britain, have all used the Delphi approach to identify clinical nursing research priorities. The procedures employed were similar. In the first round the respondents were asked to identify some areas where they believed nursing research was needed. Those most frequently indicated were returned to the respondents in subsequent rounds for re-evaluation and comments regarding the value and weighting of items.

In a Canadian study, Scherer et al (1982) successfully used the Delphi method to enable respondents to state their opinions on what constituted good quality of nursing care. The researchers concluded that it was possible to generate standards of care by using the judgments of nurse 'experts' (Farrell and Scherer, 1983). In Australia, Anderson (1986) undertook a similar research project for community nursing. In her study she used two panels of experts, the first to review and generate nursing standards and the second to evaluate the findings of the first group. Results showed an 85% consensus on 208 desirable standards.

The Delphi technique has been employed by other British nurse researchers in a variety of studies. Hitch and Murgatroyd (1983) carried out a Delphi-type survey in the North of England to uncover nurses' perceptions of and solutions to, communication problems when dealing with cancer patients. Procter (1985) also used this approach to examine the organization of care on hospital wards. She found that it could be successfully used to obtain professional consensus on the most appropriate type of care for each 'activity of living' at different patient dependency levels. White (1991) used the Delphi technique to gather the views of 102 'experts' regarding the future of psychiatric nursing.

*Attributes of the 'Delphi' for the present study*

1. The use of a panel of 'experts' for obtaining data.
2. Participants do not meet in face to face discussions.
3. The use of sequential questionnaires and/or interviews
4. The systematic emergence of a concurrence of a judgment and an opinion.
5. The guarantee of quasi-anonymity for subjects' responses.
6. The use of frequency distributions to identify patterns of agreement.
7. The use of two or more rounds between which a summary of the results of the previous round is communicated to and evaluated by panel members.

(Sackman, 1975; Strauss and Ziegler, 1975; Loughlin and Moore, 1979).

*Advantages of the Delphi technique* The advantages of the Delphi technique are well documented in the literature (Linstone and Turoff, 1975; Reid, 1988). Within this section it is proposed to concentrate on the benefits of 'Delphi' to the present study.

The Delphi process lends itself to areas of research where the aim is to identify opinions and ideological positions and to reach agreement regarding these issues (Turoff, 1970). Lindeman (1975) maintains that it is especially effective in difficult areas that can benefit from subjective judgments on a collective basis, but for which there may be no definite answer.

Perhaps the main advantage of the Delphi approach is its ability to "guide group opinion towards a final decision" (Goodman, 1987). This tendency to converge toward agreement is a unique aspect of 'Delphi' (Sackman, 1975; Loughlin and Moore, 1979) and a property considered very important to the present study.

It is well documented within the literature that, because of active 'grassroot' involvement, the consensus findings of a Delphi exercise are subject to a greater acceptance by organizational members than are decisions arrived at by other 'more direct' methods (Sackman, 1975; Loughlin and Moore, 1979). Considering the unpopularity of models among psychiatric nurses (Loughlin, 1988), perhaps the Delphi technique would bestow ward level credibility and acceptability upon any framework selected.

The findings of a Delphi operation can provide an explicit articulation from a large group of individuals concerning the direction in which the organization should be moving (Loughlin and Moore, 1979). It has also been documented that participating in a 'Delphi' survey can be a highly motivating experience for respondents (Linstone and Turoff, 1975). The feedback mechanism, where relevant material is returned to the panel members, can be a novel and interesting exercise for all concerned.

Within the literature, the Delphi technique is recognized as cost efficient (Lyons, 1981; Polit and Hungler, 1987). Even Sackman (1975) who has written an exhaustive critique on the subject admits how inexpensive it is to use, while Reid (1988) maintains that it is one of the cheapest research methods available. Charlton et al (1981) suspects that this is because only relevant and useful material is channelled back to the respondents. This avoids unnecessary 'side-tracking' and unnecessary analysis.

*Limitations of the Delphi technique* "No lesson seems to be so deeply inculcated by the experience of life as that you never trust experts...they all require to have their strong wine diluted by a very large admixture of insipid common sense." (Lord Salisbury, 1888: cited in The Oxford Dictionary of Quotations, 1988 p.413). In his

41

analysis of the Delphi method, Sackman (1975) expressed concern regarding the use of 'experts', while emphasising the possible benefits of 'non-experts'. Similarly, advocates of 'Delphi' (Linstone and Turoff, 1975), refer to the pitfall of "illusory expertise" (p. 581). A more recent critical examination of the Delphi technique noted that:

> It seems more a ppropriate to recruit individuals who have knowledge of a particular topic and who are consequently willing to engage in discussion upon it without the potentially misleading title of 'expert'. (Goodman, 1987 p.732).

Bond and Bond (1982) maintain that unlike other professions there exists no clearly identifiable clinical expert in nursing. Nonetheless, a comprehensive review of many research studies examining the role of the ward sister/charge nurse showed that he/she:

> ... emerged as the key figure within the organization and the ward team, managing, coordinating and giving care, creating the ward climate...it is mainly this grade of nurse who initiates or blocks changes in nursing practice.
> (Alexander and Orton, 1988 p.38).

Accordingly the present study identifies ward managers in long-stay psychiatric areas in Northern Ireland as possessing clinical 'expertise'. It cannot be proposed that they were 'experts' in the field of nursing models. However, from the literature it is assumed that they hold opinions and beliefs concerning, 'nursing', 'health', 'person' and 'environment' (McFarlane, 1986).

Perhaps a more important problem is the poor response rate that characterizes the final rounds of most Delphi investigations. For example, in Farrell and Scherer's research (1983) into identifying consensus on suitable nursing standards, returns were disappointing. Out of a sample of 1441 nurses, 662 agreed to participate; only 472 returned the questionnaires in round one and just 141 responded to the second round. This is a common occurrence, but seldom discussed in any report of results.

The scientific respectability of the Delphi approach has become the subject of some criticism (Sackman, 1975). However most of its proponents are aware of its scientific shortcomings. Linstone and Turoff (1975) admit that as a research approach it is more of an art than a science. According to Reid (1988), the Delphi technique caters for particular types of research questions for which a more scientific instrument may not be suitable. She notes that - as a substitute to the qualitative approach, 'Delphi' looks thoroughly scientific - as an alternative to the Likert scale it does not (Reid, 1988).

In the present study the 'Delphi' was selected strictly for exploratory purposes. Therefore the results may be what Sackman (1975) called a structured brainstorming session with responsible ward managers, as opposed to a rigid positivistic scientific exercise.

*A modified 'Delphi'* The literature describes many modifications of the basic Delphi technique (Rauch, 1979; Reid, 1988). Many of these are concerned with the creation of items, for example, the listing of different research priorities. For the present study the 'Reactive Delphi' (Weaver, 1972) was chosen as a suitable modification. As a survey method the 'Reactive Delphi' involves asking respondents to react to previously prepared information rather than generate lists of items.

*Research respondents*

These were the ward managers in long-stay psychiatric wards in Northern Ireland. Initial investigations showed that there were ninety-eight ward managers working on long-stay wards in the six psychiatric hospitals in Northern Ireland. Because this is a small number of potential respondents and the geographic distance between hospitals does not exceed eighty miles, it was decided not to sample but to pursue the entire target population.

Each of the participating hospitals was built during the last century. Similarities also extend to the types of treatment practised and the pervading influence of contemporary government policies. Out of the total number of forty nine long-stay wards, forty four had been passed for nurse training by the National Board for Nursing, Midwifery and Health Visiting for Northern Ireland. The average number of long-stay wards in each hospital was eight.

Respondents had to be registered mental nurses with complete or joint responsibility for the nursing care management on the selected wards. They had to be in full-time employment, working 37.5 hours per week or over. It was also decided to include those ward managers who work on night duty with specific responsibility for long-stay wards. In addition, it was decided to consider those who were working on rehabilitation wards. Two reasons contributed to their inclusion. Firstly, the patients within these wards meet the operational definition of long-stay patients (see above). Secondly, the literature states that most contemporary rehabilitation wards are little more than 'good long-stay wards' (Shepherd, 1984; Hume and Pullan, 1986).

Excluded from this study were those ward managers who have nursing responsibility for 'disturbed wards'. There were five such wards in Northern Ireland. The main reason for precluding this group was that many patients being cared for in these wards were acutely disturbed and did not meet the criteria of being long-stay.

*Research instruments*

Prior to collecting the data there were no published research instruments available to enable the selection of or to gauge opinions on, nursing models. Therefore to obtain the desired information it was necessary to develop new tools specifically for this study. In the interest of comprehension, the research strategy may be divided into three sections:

A.    theoretical bases instrument;
B.    model matrix instrument;
C.    semi-structured interview schedule.

*Theoretical bases instrument* It has been well documented that nursing models have their roots in one or more of the following four theories: interactional theory, behavioural theory, systems theory and developmental theory. To use this fact as a basis for model selection, concise summaries of each theory were composed.

 Personal bias was reduced by obtaining these summaries directly from the work of British nurse academics such as Chapman (1985) and McFarlane (1986). It was planned to administer them as 'single answer items': that is, requesting the respondent to choose a single item from a preselected list of alternatives. In an attempt to aid comprehension each summary was accompanied by a short elaboration. It was proposed that the respondent would choose the theory that coincides with their beliefs and attitudes regarding long-stay psychiatric patient care. This approach had the following benefits:

(1)    To identify the (seldom articulated) personal theoretical leanings of ward managers;
(2)    As a recognized strategy for model selection;
(3)    As a checking device for collaborating the subject's response to the model matrix. For example, a ward manager who advocates interactional theory would be unlikely to select model matrix statements advocating a 'system' model.

*The model matrix instrument* Since the object of this research was to enable ward managers to select an appropriate nursing model, it was necessary to expose the target population to various conceptual frameworks. There are over forty nursing models; some are too specialized, while others are only in the early stages of development. A thorough search of the literature was undertaken to discern only the most 'popular nursing models'. Nineteen such frameworks were identified using the following criteria:

1.  Each model had to be acknowledged in those professional and/or theoretical publications reviewed as a relevant conceptualization of nursing;
2.  Each model had to be recognized in the writings of at least one author (other than its originator(s)), as being practice oriented;
3.  Each model had to be identified by its originator(s) as applicable to a broad range of nursing situations.

Rather than attempt to introduce each respondent to nineteen models in their complex entirety, it was proposed to isolate the four foundational elements of 'nursing', 'health', 'person' and 'environment' from each framework. These would then be presented to the respondents as a four by nineteen 'model matrix'.

However Linstone and Turoff (1975) noted that the statements that comprise a Delphi exercise inevitably reflect the attitudes, knowledge and subjectivity of the researcher. Also the literature on decision making suggests that the wording of statements could affect choice (see chapter 3). To avoid such interpretative distortions it was consciously decided that descriptions of the four elements should be taken directly from original theoretical sources and not undergo any additional elaboration by the investigator.

The rationale behind this judgment was clear. It was felt that any attempt to simplify or to help the interviewee with terminological elucidation would introduce unnecessary bias and impose the researcher's interpretation system on the 'model statements'. In addition, by making slight differences in emphasis, real differences could be introduced in content. These factors could prejudice the respondents in their choice of model.

There is also the countercharge that non-explanation and non-elaboration may lead respondents to choose a simple yet inappropriate framework, thereby ignoring a more appropriate, although complex, framework. However, results from the pilot study showed that terminology was not a serious barrier to model selection and it was felt that the respondents in the main study could cope with the theoretical jargon. Nonetheless, to assess the effects of terminology on model selection, a question in the accompanying interview schedule relates specifically to this issue.

The 'model matrix' comprises four pages of model statements. To reduce the possibility of selection bias due to the location of the model statements each one was positioned randomly on the model matrix instrument. There was also the possibility that some ward managers may select model statements simply because they were familiar with the theorist's name. They may have been informed that a particular theorist's work would be suitable to their clinical area. To avoid this the theorist's name was omitted from the model statements and substituted with a letter from the alphabet.

*Semi-structured interview schedule* A semi-structured interview schedule was formulated. This was used to obtain additional information on whether a nurse manager would like to make an eclectic choice, why they might choose a particular model statement and in an attempt to establish the underlying opinions of the respondents towards nursing models. Of the twenty-six questions, three were open ended, thirteen were closed ended and the rest were a mixture of both. In the pursuit of thoroughness, structured prompts were developed for questions one, two, five, seven and eight

Two of the closed ended questions were of the Likert type, designed to elicit attitudes (Q 13,14) and six were concerned with demographic details such as age, sex, educational qualifications and years of service (Q 15-20). Four of the remaining closed ended questions were included in an attempt to check the authenticity of the respondents' responses to the 'model matrix' (Q 9-12). Most of the closed ended questions were 'single answer items'. Only one question (Q.19) represented a 'multiple answer item', that is, requiring the respondent to select a subset of replies from a given list.

*Reliability and validity of the research instruments* The reliability of a research instrument is concerned with the consistency or repeatability of the data collecting tool. Since the time factor militated against a 'test-retest' approach, Cronbach's Alpha was used to test the internal reliability of the interview schedule. However this test was not suitable for the open-ended items or those items that were a mixture of open and closed ended. For the closed ended questions Cronbach's alpha was .72. This indicates that the internal reliability for these questions was at an acceptable level. This does not give any indication of the reliability of the complete instrument.

The validity of a research instrument relates to the ability of the data collecting tool to test what it purports to test. Since the research tools appear to focus on the topic of investigation, namely nursing models, 'face validity' can be claimed (Treece and Treece, 1977).

Also, it has been suggested that, if research instruments are constructed from relevant literature, content validity can be claimed (Fox, 1982 p.262). This was the case with the instruments in the present study. However, in a further attempt to

46

establish content validity the instruments were sent to a panel of 13 selected nurse academics who were affiliated to institutions of higher learning throughout Great Britain. The criteria for inclusion were:

1.  The academic lectures on psychiatric nursing in tertiary educational establishments;
2.  The academic has been the author of articles/books on the utilization and implementation of nursing models.

No attempt was made at selecting this group by sampling methods. Their names, qualifications and addresses were obtained as a result of a thorough search of contemporary British theoretical and psychiatric nursing literature. They agreed that the instruments had content validity. There was no attempt to estimate the more objective 'construct validity', 'concurrent validity' or 'predictive validity' of the research instruments.

*Pilot study*

Although the target population was ward managers in long-stay psychiatric wards, eight ward sisters/charge nurses from the geriatric area of a large general hospital were used in the pilot study. It was expected that ward managers from psychogeriatric areas may have had greater similarities with the research population, however access to this group was not available at the designated time. Although 25% of the pilot group were not registered psychiatric nurses their demographic characteristics were similar to the target population. This atypical pilot group was used for the following reasons:

1.  Because of reluctance to deplete the small numbers of potential respondents for the main study, it was decided to keep the target population intact;
2.  The absence within Northern Ireland of a population of respondents similar to the target population;
3.  It was assumed that the research instruments had relevance for any area where nursing care was delivered;
4.  It was felt that the ward managers chosen for the pilot study could supply the information needed regarding the testing and administration of the research instruments;
5.  Ease of access;
6.  The pilot respondents were also involved in the care of patients on a long term basis.

After obtaining senior management approval the purposes of the pilot study were explained and anonymity and confidentiality were assured. Each respondent was encouraged to comment on their reaction to the model statements and interview questions. Comments were also sought on suitability, terminological comprehension and method of instrument administration.

*Results of the pilot study* Analysis of the pilot study findings culminated in only one question being omitted. Respondents had been asked to state whether they would like to be involved in the preliminary planning stages of model introduction. The pilot group felt that few, if any, ward sisters would answer this in the negative. Apart from minor semantic clarifications, further exclusion of research items did not arise.

Besides the information already stated, the pilot exercise also indicated how much time was required for each interview. This was on average thirty minutes. Furthermore, comments also pointed to the need for a quiet ward area to enable the respondent to concentrate on the model matrix. In conclusion, the pilot study was helpful not only regarding the practical logistics of the study, but in giving confidence to the investigator.

## Main study

Because the first part of the proposed study involved questioning nursing staff and precluded contact with patients, Ethical Committee approval was not required in this instance. The research proposal was sent to each of the four Chief Administrative Nursing Officers with a letter requesting access. They agreed to support and co-operate with the request, referring it to the relevant Directors of Nursing. After permission to proceed was granted appointments were made at the convenience of each ward manager.

For the six hospitals involved, the time spent gaining access, from initial contact with the chief administrative nursing officer to the commencement of interviews with ward managers, ranged from three weeks to two months. To save valuable time, data were collected in some Area Health Boards while waiting for other Boards to grant access.

*Anonymity and confidentiality*

Although complete anonymity appears to be a generally held principle in most Delphi surveys, Sackman (1975) argues that this can lead to a lack of accountability for the views expressed. According to Goodman (1987) it encourages hasty ill-considered judgments. In an attempt to avoid this problem, some researchers, including Rauch (1979) favour 'quasi-anonymity'. This implies that the respondents may be known to one another, but their judgments and opinions remain strictly anonymous. Rauch

48

postulates that knowing who the other respondents are should have the effect of motivating the panelists to participate.

In the present study, each respondent was aware that his or her clinical counterparts would also be surveyed. This was inevitable considering the parochial nature of the hospitals concerned and the dual ward manager system in many wards. Therefore the idea of 'quasi-anonymity' was adopted. However, as a safeguard, the importance of respondents not discussing their responses with others was stressed both in verbal and written communications.

Respondents were given an assurance of complete confidentiality. They were informed that no hospital, ward or individual would be identifiable in any report or publication.

*The data collection procedure*

This took place between May 1987 and August 1987. For ease of description the data collecting process will be divided into two main sections:

A.    theoretical bases;
      model matrix (Round one);
      semi-structured interview;

B.    model matrix (Round two).

The theoretical bases instrument, the model matrix instrument (round one) and the semi-structured interview schedule were presented to the respondents using a face to face interview format. To maintain a high degree of conformity across interviews all probes and prompts were preplanned and prerecorde.

Following preliminary introductions with each respondent, the nature of the study and the assurance of confidentiality were reemphasized. A verbal account was given of what nursing models were and how they differed from the nursing process. It was stressed that apart from granting access, nursing administration was not involved in the planning, execution or evaluation of the project. Respondents were also informed that it would take approximately thirty minutes to complete the research instrument. After ensuring that there would be minimal upheaval of the care setting the interview was conducted on a quiet area of the ward. More often than not this was the ward office.

*Theoretical bases instrument* As outlined above this instrument incorporated synoptic outlines of the four main theoretical foundations of nursing models. Each synopsis was accompanied by the short structured elaboration. Once it was decided that the respondent understood the content, they were instructed to study each theoretical outline. They were then asked to tick the one that best reflected their views and beliefs concerning long-stay psychiatric patient care.

*The model matrix (round one)* As stated earlier, the model matrix comprised nineteen anonymous 'model statements', each pertaining to how individual nursing models viewed nursing, health, person and environment. The respondents were asked to read each one carefully, making a first and second choice of those that they believed to be suitable for the nursing care of the long-stay psychiatric patient. They were informed that they had to choose a model statement in its entirety. The respondent's first option was indicated with a 'tick' in the box provided and a note was taken of their second choice. Each respondent was given an opportunity (if they so desired) to change their mind and reselect.

*Semi-structured interview* The design and content of this instrument have been described above. It was presented to the respondent immediately following the administration of the model matrix. Once the respondents had chosen their preferred first and second model statements, question one in the interview schedule asked if they would like to modify their choice by selecting nursing, health, person and environment from different unconnected model statements. In this way respondents had the opportunity to form an eclectic model statement.

With questions one, two, five, seven and eight, a list of alternatives were read from a prompt card. It was stressed to all respondents that they must be as accurate and as honest in their replies as possible.

Bias was avoided in the interview situation by ensuring that there was consistency in the method of question delivery; every interview was conducted in much the same way, including the ordering of prompts and elaborations. According to Powell (1982), "the greater the social distance between the researcher and the respondents, the less adequate the communication between them." (p.36). Because the investigator was of the same organizational rank as the interviewees, he was familiar with what Powell called the 'native language'. This limited the possibility of misunderstanding the respondent's meaning.

*Response rate for round one* In round one of this two round Delphi operation, responses were obtained from ninety-five respondents. This represents a response rate of 96.9% (See table 4.1). Three ward managers were on prolonged sick leave.

50

**Table 4.1. Number of long-stay psychiatric wards and number of staff who responded in each of the six hospitals**

| Hospital | Long-Stay Wards | Respondent Numbers |
|----------|-----------------|--------------------|
| A | 12 | 25 |
| B | 8 | 15 |
| C | 7 | 13 |
| D | 6 | 13 |
| E | 8 | 16 |
| F | 8 | 13 |
| Total    6 | 49 | 95 |

The high response rate may be the result of four factors. Firstly, the respondents could relate to the investigator who, like themselves, was a psychiatric charge nurse (although seconded to undertake research). Secondly, respondents were pleased that someone "was at last asking for their opinions". Thirdly, the respondents believed that the subject matter was relevant to the future of their practice. Finally, it is possible that since they were originally informed of the study by senior nurses, respondents may have associated refusal to participate with management censure.

*model matrix (round two)* Those 'model statements' that were favoured by most respondents in the first round ( > 51% ), were returned to each respondent in a one page postal questionnaire. A similar strategy was used by Murgatroyd and Hitch (1984) and Anderson (1986). The accompanying letter requested that the respondents reconsider carefully the presented alternatives and rank them according to their preference, taking into account the needs of long-stay psychiatric patient care. Such ranking of items is a common feature of most Delphi exercises (Goodman, 1986).

A section of the instrument was set aside for comments and respondents were again asked not to discuss their choice with others. Furthermore, since it was believed that no additional relevant information could be obtained from the theoretical bases section and the interview schedule, it was decided to exclude these instruments from the second round of the 'Delphi'.

The literature contains many references to the disadvantages of the postal questionnaire format (Diers, 1979; Nachmias and Nachmias, 1981). Nevertheless for the present study it was seen as a useful method for distributing round two of the 'Delphi'. This was because of the following reasons:

1.  The respondents were already familiar with the content of the research instrument and therefore the prospect of misinterpretation was low;
2.  Because it could not be foreseen how many rounds would be required for consensus, an inexpensive method of instrument distribution had to be considered;
3.  The respondents could examine the alternative model statements at length prior to responding.

*Response rate for round two* There was a return rate of 100% in round two. This is highly unusual not only with the Delphi technique, but also with conventional postal questionnaires. The following factors may have contributed to the high response: the inclusion of a stamped self addressed envelope, the respondents knew the researcher from the previous interview - thereby appreciating the 'personal touch', the respondents were aware that the second round was formulated from their prior responses - hence they realized that they were an integral part of the project and follow up of five late responses resulted in the reissuing and eventual return of instruments. The follow-up procedure involved telephone contact to ask non-respondents if they had received or misplaced the research correspondence.

*Data analysis plan*

The data were coded in a form that would ease analysis using the CSM 20/4-VAX computer at the University of Ulster. Sub programmes from the Statistical Package for the Social Sciences (SPSS$^x$) (Nie et al, 1970), were suitable for all aspects of the data analysis.

The data analysis plan involved analysing the quantitative data using mostly descriptive statistics. The qualitative data obtained from items one, two, five, seven, eight and twenty-one of the semi-structured interview schedule were confirmed with the respondents at the time of interview. Later they were analysed using modified content analysis to categorize the comments. An experienced psychiatric nurse, external to the study, was employed to assist in this task. He independently post-coded responses into categories and these were compared with the categorizations made by the researcher. There were only four areas of disagreement and these were discussed and reassessed by both reviewers before a final decision was made.

In comparing the respondent's choice of model according to their demographic details and their opinions towards models, cross tabulations and the non-parametric Chi Square test were used to examine how much weight can be placed on identified relationships. These will be described as 'significant' where they could have occurred by chance not more than five times in one hundred (P < .05). Cramer's V test was applied to the results to gauge the strength of any significant relationship.

# 5 Presentation of findings

This chapter presents the findings obtained from applying the three research tools discussed in chapter four. The results will be presented in the following manner:

1. An outline of the demographic characteristics of the respondents;
2. A statement of each individual research question;
3. Presentation of the data related to each research question.

**Characteristics of respondents**

The respondents consisted of ninety five ward managers from forty nine long-stay wards in the province's six psychiatric hospitals. The gender distribution among the ward managers was fifty two males (54.7%) and forty three females (45.3%).

*General education*

**Figure 5.1. General educational attainment of respondents**

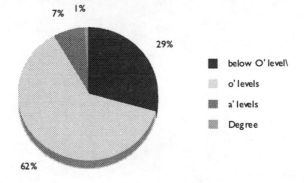

Figure 5.1 indicates that most of the respondents (62.1%) had obtained a general educational equivalent to 'O' level standard.

*Nursing qualifications*

All respondents possessed the Registered Mental Nursing (R.M.N) qualification. If this qualification is excluded from the data, the State Registered Nursing (S.R.N.) qualification emerges as the mode with a frequency of thirty seven (38.9%).

**Figure 5.2. Distribution of respondents in terms of nursing qualifications**

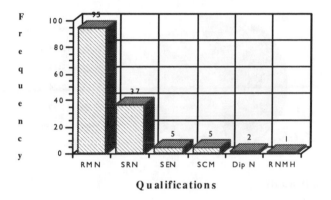

*Age*

The distribution of age in this population mimics a normal Gaussian distribution. Therefore the arithmetic mean and standard deviation can be used as measures of central tendency and variability respectively. The mean age of the population was 45.3 years with a standard deviation of 18.73 years.

**Figure 5.3. Distribution of respondents in terms of age**

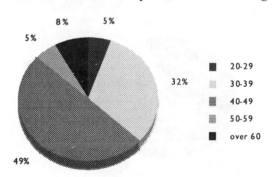

*Years in nursing*

Figure 5.4 shows the number of years respondents spent in nursing, excluding those years spent in nurse training. The median is 23.9 years with a semi interquartile range of 5.8 years. Sixty four respondents had been nursing between fifteen and thirty years, nine for less than fifteen years and twenty two for thirty or more years.

**Figure 5.4. Number of years respondents have spent in nursing (excluding training)**

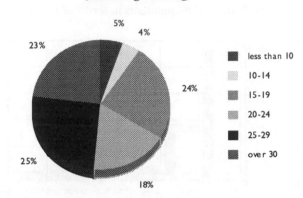

*Years in long-stay wards*

The median number of years respondents spent nursing on long-stay wards has been calculated as 6.2 years with a semi interquartile range of 4. Seventeen have worked in this specialty for two years or less, while fifty one have been employed there on a continuous basis for six years or more.

**Figure 5.5. Distribution of respondents in terms of number of years continuously working in long-stay areas**

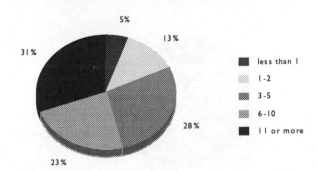

## Findings from the theroetical bases instrument

*Research question*

What theoretical basis do ward managers favour for nursing practice on long-stay psychiatric wards in Northern Ireland?

### Figure 5.6. Distribution of respondents according to their choice of theoretical base

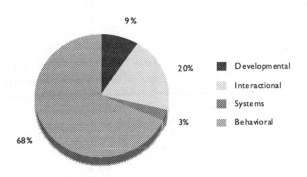

The behavioural theory was the most popular choice of theoretical base with sixty four respondents (67.4%) opting for it. Nineteen respondents (20%) selected the Interactional Theory. Nine respondents chose Developmental theory. Three respondents (3.2%) believed that Systems theory best suited their clinical requirements.

## Findings from the model matrix instrument

*Research question*

What nursing model (from a predetermined list of options) will the majority of ward managers in long-stay psychiatric areas select as suitable for their particular patient care group?

This research question represented the dominant focus of this part of the study. As alluded to above, the central philosophies from nineteen (anonymous) nursing models were distributed and redistributed in the form of a 'model matrix' to ninety five ward managers using a two part 'Delphi' exercise. Each respondent was asked to select a first and second choice of an appropriate nursing model. The results of round one of the 'Delphi' are shown in table 5.1.

**Table 5.1. Distribution of respondents by their preferred first and second choice of nursing model**

| Nursing Model Title | Frequency of Selection (n = 95) | | |
| --- | --- | --- | --- |
| | 1st Choice | 2nd Choice | Total Score (points) |
| Minshull et al | 25 | 12 | 62 |
| Roper et al | 19 | 15 | 49 |
| Henderson | 10 | 20 | 40 |
| Orem | 8 | 8 | 24 |
| King | 8 | 5 | 21 |
| Travelbee | 8 | 3 | 19 |
| Orlando | 6 | 7 | 19 |
| Riehl | 3 | 4 | 10 |
| Levine | 2 | 4 | 8 |
| Wiedenbach | 2 | 2 | 6 |
| Peplau | 0 | 6 | 6 |
| Newman | 1 | 2 | 4 |
| Rogers | 1 | 2 | 4 |
| ROY | 1 | 0 | 2 |
| Neuman | 1 | 0 | 2 |
| Fitzpatrick | 0 | 2 | 2 |
| Johnson | 0 | 1 | 1 |
| Patterson & Zderad | 0 | 1 | 1 |
| Parse | 0 | 0 | 0 |
| Total | 95 | 95 | 276 |

During analysis of this data a first choice was awarded two points whereas a second choice was awarded one point. As demonstrated in table 5.1 the Human Needs model (HNM) of Minshull et al (1986) achieved a total of sixty two points, Roper et al's Activities of Living model (1980) scored forty nine points and Henderson's Activities of Daily Living model (1966) obtained forty points. These three models all have their roots in Behavioural theory.

*Round two 'Delphi'*

Those model statements favoured by the majority of Frespondents in the first round (> 51%) of the 'Delphi' were returned to each respondent in the second round. Since the models of Minshull et al, Roper et al and Henderson received 56.8% of the first preference choices and 54.7% of the overall score, it was decided to redistribute these three frameworks to each respondent in the form of a postal questionnaire. Respondents were asked to rank each of the three models according to preference. Once again the identity of the theorists was kept anonymous. The results of this iteration are shown in figure 5.7.

**Figure 5.7. Frequencies of first, second and third choices of appropriate nursing models by respondents**

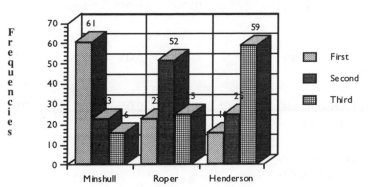

As shown in figure 5.7. most respondents selected Minshull et al's Human Needs model as their first choice with Roper et al's Activities of Living and Henderson's Activities of Daily Living models coming second and third respectively.

An alternative analytical strategy was to award a first choice - three points, a second choice - two points and a third choice - one point. The results of this approach revealed that Minshull et al's model received 232 points, Roper et al's model received 188 points and Henderson's model received 150 points.

**Relationship between choice of nursing model and demographic profile of respondent**

*Research question*

Is there a relationship between choice of model and demographic profile of the ward manager (age, sex, length of time in psychiatric nursing, length of time in long-stay wards, nursing qualifications, educational standard)?

The relationship between the respondents' choice of model in the second round of the 'Delphi' and their demographic profile was examined. Due to the fact that the data were nominal in nature, the non-parametric Chi Square test was used to establish whether relationships were significant. In addition, Cramer's V test was applied to discover the strength of the relationship. The results are shown in table 5.2.

### Table 5.2. Relationships between demographic profile of respondents and their preferred choice of nursing model

| Relationship | df | Chi Sq | p | signif | Cramer's V |
|---|---|---|---|---|---|
| Choice of model by age | 4 | 10.39 | 0.05 | yes | .19 |
| Choice of model by sex | 2 | 6.23 | 0.05 | yes | .12 |
| Choice of model by education | 2 | 4.16 | 0.05 | no | .01 |
| Choice of model by qualifications | 2 | 1.51 | 0.05 | no | .001 |
| Choice of model by years in nursing | 2 | 2.98 | 0.05 | no | .01 |
| Choice of model by years in long-stay wards | 2 | 3.89 | 0.05 | no | .01 |

Results of the Chi Square test showed that most of the respondents' demographic data had no significant impact on their choice of model. Although the variables sex and age had a statistically significant influence, Cramer's V demonstrated that the strength of the influence was almost negligible. Furthermore as two tailed non-directional hypotheses were used, the direction of the significance cannot be specified.

**Findings from interview schedule**

*Evidence of eclectic tendencies*

In order to see if a pattern of eclecticism existed in the respondents' choice of model, an opportunity was given for them to construct a 'hybrid' model statement. To do this they were allowed to select the individual elements nursing, health, person and environment from whatever part of the model matrix they wished. This enabled them to formulate a personal eclectic model statement.

Twenty six respondents (27%) took the opportunity to do this. Although they could select all four elements from different models most decided to modify their original choice by changing only one element. Of the nine respondents who had originally selected a developmental model statement, four (44%) wanted to modify the elements within it: of the 19 who had selected an interactional model statement ten (52%) wanted to modify the elements; and of the sixty four who had selected a behavioural model statement, twelve (19%) wanted to modify the elements. None of the three respondents who had opted for a system model statement wanted to change their initial selection.

The essential elements from the behavioural model statements were the most popular alternative selections. Of the thirty two changes made twenty (63%) related to elements from behavioural models; seven (22%) related to elements from interactional models; four (13%) related to elements from developmental models and one (3%) related to an element from a system model. Results also indicate that the behavioural model located at code 5/H was a popular alternative source of elements. This was Minshull et al's (1986) model.

Although this was an interesting exercise, the number of respondents who wished to modify their initial selection is too small for the detection of an overall eclectic pattern. However, this activity does indicate that when given the opportunity of selecting essential elements for a nursing model, 27% of the respondents favoured an eclectic perspective.

*Respondents' views regarding nursing, health, person and environment*

A series of closed-ended questions within the interview schedule concentrated on establishing what the respondents' personal views were concerning health, nursing, person and environment. Statements regarding these concepts were formulated from the main nursing model philosophies and were presented to the respondents as a means of validating their choice of model statement from the model matrix. In order to encourage a focused decision each respondent was restricted to a single choice. Their responses are outlined in tables 5.3 - 5.6.

**Table 5.3. Distribution of respondents by their choice of prepared
statements on what is Health**

| Health is; | Frequency of Response | |
|---|---|---|
| | Number (n=95) | Percentage |
| Biopsychosocial well-being | 44 | 46.3 |
| Mental & physical comfort | 16 | 16.8 |
| State of wellness & illness | 13 | 13.7 |
| Optimum independence | 10 | 10.5 |
| State of wholeness | 8 | 8.4 |
| Positive adapting to stresses | 4 | 4.2 |
| Total | 95 | 100.0 |

**Table 5.4. Distribution of respondents by their choice of prepared
statements on what is the Person**

| The Person is; | Frequency of Response | |
|---|---|---|
| | Number (n=95) | Percentage |
| One who is always learning | 34 | 35.8 |
| A whole person with basic needs | 22 | 23.2 |
| A biopsychosocial individual | 18 | 18.9 |
| One who can adapt to change | 17 | 17.9 |
| An open system | 4 | 4.2 |
| Total | 95 | 100.0 |

**Table 5.5. Distribution of respondents by their choice of prepared statements on what is Nursing**

| Nursing is; | Frequency of Response | |
| --- | --- | --- |
| | Number (n=95) | Percentage |
| Helping towards independence | 69 | 72.6 |
| An interpersonal process | 16 | 16.8 |
| Concerned with human interaction | 6 | 6.3 |
| Helping patient adapt to stresses | 2 | 2.1 |
| Intervention to prevent ill-health | 2 | 2.1 |
| Total | 95 | 100.0 |

**Table 5.6. Distribution of respondents by their choice of prepared statements on what is the Environment**

| The Environment is; | Frequency of Response | |
| --- | --- | --- |
| | Number (n=95) | Percentage |
| The area where man functions | 47 | 49.5 |
| A system interacting with person | 29 | 30.5 |
| An internal & external condition | 13 | 13.7 |
| A constraining/sustaining force | 5 | 5.3 |
| An internal part of the person | 1 | 1.1 |
| Total | 95 | 100.0 |

*Reasons for model choice*

The researcher was interested in discovering what factors influenced the respondents in their choice of nursing model from the 'model matrix'. A series of structured prompts accompanied this question. Results are shown in table 5.7.

63

**Table 5.7. Factors which influenced respondents in their selection of a
nursing model from the 'model matrix'**

| Influencing Factors. | Frequency of response<br>Number   (n = 95) |
|---|---|
| Suits respondent's patient care group | 40 |
| Suits respondent's own views | 40 |
| Suits respondent's ward | 34 |
| Wording used | 9 |
| Possesses flexibility | 9 |
| Total number of influencing factors | 132 |

*Familiarity with models of nursing*

Fifty eight respondents (61%) stated that they had read 'something' in the nursing press concerning models of nursing while thirty seven respondents (38.9%) had never read anything on nursing models.  In addition, eight respondents had been unaware of the existence of nursing models whilst eighty seven respondents (91.6%) had heard about them. As a follow up question, the researcher asked the latter respondents of what models they had heard. Their responses are shown in table 5.8.

**Table 5.8. Nursing models with which respondents were  familiar**

| Nursing Model | Frequency of Responses<br>Number (n =87) |
|---|---|
| Roper et al | 65 |
| Orem | 54 |
| Henderson | 21 |
| Roy | 8 |
| Riehl | 7 |
| Rogers | 5 |
| Johnson | 2 |
| Peplau | 1 |
| Total number of responses | 163 |

*Information from nurse management*

When asked what information about nursing models had respondents received from nursing administration, Fifty eight respondents (61.1%) replied that they had received some, while thirty seven respondents stated they had received none whatsoever. The type of information the former respondents received is presented in table 5.9.

**Table 5.9. Type of information concerning nursing models received by respondents from their nursing hierarchy**

| Type of Information | Frequency of Response Numbers (n=58) |
|---|---|
| Reading material to ward | 41 |
| Inservice training | 26 |
| Ward meetings | 5 |
| Total number of responses | 72 |

Over seventy percent of those respondents who had received information from nursing administration stated that it took the form of photocopied journal articles distributed to the wards via the internal mail system or handed in by nursing officers. Twenty six respondents had attended inservice training days where "models were mentioned". Five respondents in one hospital had participated in unit meetings specifically set up to discuss nursing models. No respondent had been offered or had received information from personnel in nurse education.

*The use of nursing models at ward level*

Sixty five respondents (68.4%) stated that they had never consciously used a model of nursing on their wards, while thirty respondents (31.6%) claimed that they were using a model of nursing on their ward at the time of interview (June/July 1988). When this latter group was asked to identify the frameworks they were using, they gave the following responses (See figure 5.8.)

# Figure 5.8. Nursing models which were stated as being used by respondents (n=30)

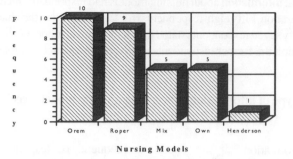

As shown in figure 5.8. Orem's model was claimed as being used more often than any other. Five respondents said that they used a "mixture of Orem and Roper". Five other respondents claimed that they used their own model. Henderson's Activities of Daily Living framework was said to be used by one respondent.

*Implementation problems with nursing models*

The researcher was interested in finding out if the respondents saw any potential problems with the implementation of a nursing model. Sixty six respondents (69.5%) believed that problems would arise while twenty three respondents (24.2%) maintained that they could foresee no problems. Six respondents (6.3%) were undecided as to whether problems would arise or not. The researcher asked those respondents who anticipated implementation problems to outline the factors they considered potentially problematic. Their responses are presented in table 5.10.

## Table 5.10. Factors identified by respondents as potential problems areas

| Anticipated Problem | Frequency of Response Numbers (n = 66) |
|---|---|
| Type of patient mix on ward | 16 |
| Practical application | 15 |
| Lack of staff knowledge | 14 |
| Staff movement | 10 |
| Staff numbers | 6 |
| Lack of managerial support | 5 |
| Total number of anticipated problems | 66 |

66

As shown in Table 5.10 sixteen respondents believed that because patients on long-stay wards differed greatly in terms of age, diagnosis and nursing care requirements, proper implementation of a nursing model would be difficult. Fifteen respondents maintained that practical problems such as writing skills and documentation could be potential stumbling blocks to successful implementation. Thirty responses were staff related; fourteen pertained to the ignorance of staff towards models of nursing, ten concerned the practice of moving staff from ward to ward and six regarded staffing levels. Five maintained that without management support nursing models would not be introduced correctly at ward level.

*Preparation required for model implementation*

Respondents were asked what preparation ward managers required prior to the implementation of nursing models in their areas. Table 5.11. illustrates their responses to this question.

**Table 5.11. Type of preparation respondents say they require prior to the introduction of nursing models at ward level**

| Preparation Required | Frequency of Response Numbers (n = 95) |
|---|---|
| Workshops | 53 |
| See the model in action | 37 |
| Reading material | 20 |
| Talk to those who use it | 11 |
| Open discussion | 7 |
| Formal lectures | 7 |
| | |
| Total number of responses | 135 |

All respondents felt strongly that some type of preparation was necessary if ward based nurses were to implement nursing models properly. Most respondents stated that workshops should be arranged where nursing staff can acquire practical experience in the handling of documentation and assessment procedures. The next best type of preparation was concerned with seeing the model working. Only a minority felt that open discussions and formal lectures were useful methods of preparation. Many pointed out that written information received at lectures was filed away and seldom referred to again.

67

## Opinions reharding models of nursing

*Research question*

What are the opinions of ward managers on long-stay psychiatric wards in Northern Ireland towards nursing models?

Respondents were asked to specify their level of agreement with the statement that nursing models were an American 'fad'. Their responses are shown in figure 5.9.

**Figure 5.9. Distribution of respondents' responses as to whether nursing models are an American 'fad'**

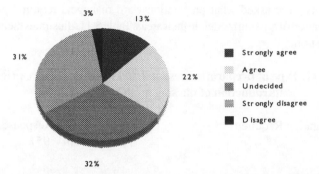

The three broad response categories of agreement, disagreement and indecision received a similar number of responses each. The researcher then asked respondents to state their level of agreement/disagreement on the statement that nursing models were useful tools for the practice of nursing care. Their responses are illustrated in figure 5.10.

**Figure 5.10. Distribution of respondents' responses as to whether nursing models are useful tools for nursing practice**

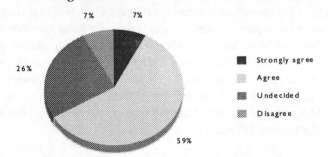

Most respondents concurred with the statement while a small minority disagreed. A substantial number of respondents were undecided as to how they viewed the statement.

The final question on the interview schedule was open ended and required respondents to clearly and honestly state their overall opinion regarding models of nursing. With the help of an experienced psychiatric nurse, external to the study, the responses were post coded into four main categories represented in figure 5.11.

**Figure 5.11. Distribution of respondents' opinions concerning nursing models**

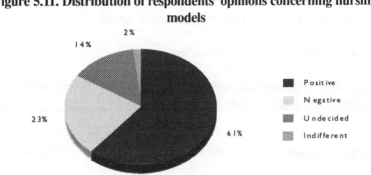

As shown in figure 5.11. the majority of respondents put forward an opinion which was positive in nature. Approximately a quarter of all respondents voiced negative views. Although a small number of respondents said they were undecided two respondents stated that they "could not care either way". None of the respondents gave a mixed view. Those perceptions which were positive in content are specified in table 5.12.

**Table 5.12. Positive views on nursing models put forward by respondents**

| Positive Opinions | Frequency of Response Number (n = 58) |
|---|---|
| Raises quality of patient care | 20 |
| Systematic method of care delivery | 20 |
| Helps students | 6 |
| Fits in with nursing process | 5 |
| Individualizes care | 5 |
| Adds a psychosocial perspective | 2 |
| Total number of positive responses | 58 |

69

Table 5.12 indicates that a popular view held by respondents concerned the positive effect that nursing models had on quality of care and method of care delivery. Examples of respondents' positive comments include:

Models may be good at getting people to wake up to what they should be doing.

Models will help us improve our standards of care.

They are useful for student teaching.

Models just don't look at the physical care of patients.

It should make the nursing process easier.

Although only a minority of respondents (23.1%) viewed nursing models negatively they tended to be more vociferous in their statements

### Table 5.13. Negative views on nursing models put forward by respondents

| Negative Opinions | Frequency of Response Numbers (n = 22) |
|---|---|
| A. WORK RELATED; | |
| Too much writing | 10 |
| Too constraining | 3 |
| Complicates caring | 2 |
| Models mean extra work | 2 |
| Management ploy | 2 |
| B. MODEL RELATED; | |
| Too many | 6 |
| Own models are fine | 6 |
| Too idealistic | 3 |
| Past was better | 2 |
| Value limited to user | 2 |

## C. APPLICATION;

| | |
|---|---|
| Need a suitable one | 7 |
| Models need to be tested | 5 |
| Nurses need educating | 5 |
| Models must be flexible | 4 |
| Need increased resources | 3 |
| Need management support | 1 |
| | |
| Total number of negative responses | 63 |

Table 5.13. shows that the negative views of respondents regarding nursing models tended to emphasize the extra work involved, the inherent inappropriateness of many models and the problems with using them in practice. Examples of negative comments include:

In the past nurses did it and didn't write about it, now I suspect they write about it but don't do it.

Is Roper one ? - I seem to remember that rubbish!

An additional concept to complement the disaster of the nursing process.

All these new fangled ideas that emerge from America are wrecking nursing here.

Models are just the vehicles for some people to make a name for themselves.

It's okay for ivory tower academics to come up with these frameworks but I work in the real world; unlike them I see the problems for which there is little that can be done.

**Relationship between choice of nursing model and respondents' opinions**

*Research question*

Is there a relationship between choice of nursing model and positive and/or negative opinions towards nursing models?

The relationship between respondents' choice of model in the second round of the

71

'Delphi' and whether they held a positive or negative opinion towards nursing models was examined. Once again the Chi Square and Cramer's V tests were used. Results are shown in table 5.14.

**Table 5.14. Relationships between respondents' positive and negative opinions and their preferred choice of nursing model**

| Relationship | df | Chi Sq | p | signif | Cramer's V |
|---|---|---|---|---|---|
| Choice of model by negative opinions | 2 | 3.25 | 0.05 | no | .03 |
| Choice of model by positive opinions | 2 | 2.73 | 0.05 | no | .03 |

Table 5.14 shows that according to the Chi Square test the relationship between choice of nursing model and both positive and negative opinions is not significant at the 0.05 level of significance. Similarly, the use of Cramer's V shows that the strength of any perceived relationship is very small at 0.03 (Normal V range = 0 - 1).

# 6 Discussion of findings

## Introduction

An attempt will be made in this chapter to interpret the results outlined in the previous chapter. To highlight aspects relevant to the discussion, statements obtained from the research respondents will be included in the text. Further, an attempt will be made to emphasize the possible limitations of the research instruments and the research approach.

It is proposed to structure the discussion section around the three research instruments employed. Emphasis will also be placed on the responses obtained to the research questions.

### Theoretical bases

The fact that sixty four (67.4%) respondents selected behavioural theory as a suitable conceptual basis for long-stay psychiatric nursing practice seems to support Hardy's (1986) assertion that nursing is a behavioural science. Behaviourally based nursing models are founded on the proposition that human beings are normally able to function by their own efforts, meeting their own needs, carrying out their own 'activities of living' and fulfilling their own 'self care' requirements (Glasper, 1990). Results show that most of the ward managers surveyed favoured this theoretical philosophy for their patients.

Since interaction with patients has been seen as encapsulating 'what psychiatric nursing is all about' (Powell, 1982), one may have expected many more respondents to favour the interactional theory. However only eighteen (20%) ward managers did so. One possible reason for its lack of popularity may be because when they were student nurses the respondents did not receive in-depth instruction in the necessary interactional skills and so do not practice nurse patient interaction to any great extent. This fact has been emphasized in the research of Altschul (1972) and Towell (1975).

Systems theory was the least popular of the theories presented. Only 3 (3%) of those ward managers questioned felt it was an appropriate way of viewing long-stay psychiatric patient care. Many respondents found it "very mechanical" or "too akin to medicine", a view shared by Grahame (1987).

Developmental theory concentrates on the individual's stage, direction and potential for human growth and maturation. It was seen as appropriate by 9 (9%) of the ward managers. Considering its psychiatric origins and because it has been the 'foundation stone' for the psychiatric nursing frameworks of Peplau (1952) and Travelbee (1966), one may have expected it to be selected by more respondents. Perhaps a reason why this did not occur was because many patients in long-stay psychiatric wards were elderly and dependent and, as Carson et al (1989) found, ward staff link this with steady deterioration rather than developmental potential and positive change.

It appears therefore that the respondents could select a theoretical approach which they believed was suitable to their work. In her research Altschul (1972) searched in vain for evidence of any theoretical principles that appeared to guide psychiatric nurses in their work with patients. McIlwaine (1980) believed Altschul's lack of success was because at the time of her study British psychiatric nurses had little or no knowledge regarding conceptual approaches to patient care. Fifteen years later the situation has changed. Results from this present study indicate that fifty seven (61%) of those ward managers surveyed said they had read articles in the nursing press on conceptual frameworks in nursing, while eighty seven (91.6%) were aware of their existence. Perhaps psychiatric nurses today are better equipped to identify and state their theoretical leanings.

*Model choice ('Delphi' round one)*

Meleis (1985) devised a tripartite classificatory system for models of nursing:

Category A.    Those that describe what nurses 'do';
Category B.    Those that describe the 'how' of nursing;
Category C.    Those that describe the 'why' of nursing.

The model selections made by respondents in the first round of the 'Delphi' fitted Meleis's classifications almost perfectly. In other words those models that received the greatest number of responses tended to relate to category A, those which received

74

a 'medium' response relate to category B and those which received a weak or a non response relate to category C.

*Models that received a good response* Results highlighted in the previous chapter show that in the first round of the 'Delphi' the respondent's most popular preference was the 'Human Needs' model (HNM) of Minshull et al (1986); the second most popular choice was the 'Activities Of Living' model of Roper et al (1985) and the third most popular choice was the 'Activities of Daily Living' model of Henderson (1966). On average they received eighteen first preference responses each. One can ask why most respondents selected these three models. There are many possible reasons for this.

These models are comparable because they tend to describe what nurses do rather than the how or why of nursing care: and indeed many of those surveyed, saw themselves as the 'doers' rather than the 'conceptualists' of nursing care. This perception of their role was expressed by the following statements:

> Students today are more interested in writing, than they are in doing.

> They can order us to use a particular model but we are the ones that have to do the work.

Secondly, although respondents were not made aware what theoretical base a particular 'model statement' belonged to, the top three choices were all behavioural models. To a large extent this had been previously indicated by the results from the 'theoretical bases' instrument. This gives an amount of credence to Aggelton and Chalmer's (1986) assertion that by studying the theoretical foundations of models, nurses could make some preliminary decisions about the type of framework which is most appropriate to their patient care group.

The three models selected are concerned with the maintenance of independence and the avoidance of dependence for basic human needs. They all relate to Maslow's 'Hierarchy Of Needs' with Henderson (1966) and Roper et al (1985) both focusing heavily on the area of physiological needs. To an extent Roper et al's model is largely an anglicized version of Henderson's work. Each concentrates on the individual's ability to be independent in those activities which we must all practise to have an optimum quality of life.

In Northern Ireland's psychiatric hospitals most 'good' long-stay patients have been transferred to rehabilitation areas or to the community. As a result many of those remaining in long-stay areas are over sixty five years of age and often dependent. In addition, approximately 20% of long-stay psychiatric patients in the province suffer from some form of mental handicap. Perhaps therefore, it was not surprising that models concentrating on independence in basic human needs were favoured by nurse managers looking after such individuals. Several respondents stated that:

> The majority of our long-stay patients are elderly. First of all they need help with their basic daily activities not 'highfalutin' social skills work.

This has been highlighted in other psychiatric nursing research studies. For example, Powell (1982) found that nurse training in one British psychiatric hospital focused on 'assisting patients in achieving the optimal level of independence for daily living activities within their own individual capabilities'. Cormack (1983), who researched the role of the psychiatric nurse in Scotland, observed that the nurse's function in long-stay wards centred around 'staff-initiated therapeutic intervention' in an attempt to reestablish the patients' basic independence skills.

Of all the nursing model statements presented to the research population these three frameworks retain the closest links with the medical model. Their popularity among the respondents reflects the huge input medical ideology has had on psychiatric nursing over the years. Results show that eighty six (90.5%) respondents have spent fifteen or more years, exclusive of training, as psychiatric nurses. Therefore many of them have had their education and experience based upon the medical model as described in Nolan's study (1989).

Thirty seven (38.9%) of the ward managers surveyed possessed a General Nursing qualification. This implies that they had undergone in-depth training in the physical aspects of nursing care. It is tempting to suggest that this experience may have had an influence on their choice of model. Results show that twenty three of these respondents, representing 62.2% of their number, selected a behavioural model. However, although this appears consequential, statistical analysis of model choice with qualification indicates a non significant relationship.

Although at the time of selection the respondents were unaware of it, two out of the three models selected were British. This was an interesting outcome considering that most of the models presented were American. This may lead one to suspect that the terminology used in various models had, either positively or negatively, influenced their choice. However responses to the interview schedule suggest that this was not so. When each respondent was asked to state what effect 'wording' had on their selection of an appropriate model only nine ward managers (9%) felt that it had any impact at all. However it is possible that at a subconscious level terminology may have had an effect.

Perhaps their unknowing selection of British nursing models was indeed relevant, befitting our Western European view of patient care. In 1986 McFarlane asked if American models were transferable to nursing practice in Britain and Girot (1990) argues that the application of American nursing models to British nursing practice is not always appropriate. It has also been widely recognized that nursing models from the United States have their roots in a different culture, a different health care structure, different values and beliefs and a different nurse training scheme.

Correspondingly, Cowan (1986) writes that Roper et al's model (1985) is simple to understand, an observation that may equally be applied to the work of Minshull et al (1986) and Henderson (1966). The basic concepts inherent in their work are uncomplicated and comprehensible, personifying both 'parsimony' and 'Occam's Razor'. Experiences with the nursing process have encouraged a feeling of scepticism among many psychiatric nurses regarding 'academic innovations'. Perhaps therefore a simple model holds certain attractions to the busy practitioner. The utilization of a simple model does much to allay fears, because such a model would be easily understood and therefore non threatening.

Although Orem's (1980) 'Self Care' framework is also concerned with 'what nurses do' only eight ward managers believed it was a suitable model on which to base their practice. To a large extent their rejection of it is echoed in the literature. Collister (1986) maintains that Orem's work has proved difficult to use in psychiatry both as an assessment tool and as a guide to formulating patient care goals. Smith (1986) recognized its potential unacceptability among psychiatric nurses:

> For many psychiatric nurses the notion that patients should be encouraged to self care along the lines suggested by Orem generates incredulity and disbelief giving rise to visions of anarchy and chaos in hospital wards. (p.71).

The 'Self Care' framework, because of its inclusion within psychiatric nurse training curricula, is being promoted as the model of choice for long-stay psychiatric practice in Northern Ireland. Ward managers in these areas claim that they have been overtly and covertly encouraged to use it:

> If student nurses coming onto this ward must write a care study based on Orem's model, then we must use Orem here.

> I hear tell Orem's the one we will be using.

Considering the lack of support for Orem's model among the respondents and with many psychiatric nursing authors, it is perhaps worrying that it may be unquestionably assimilated into clinical psychiatric nursing practice. Such a move, if it proves injudicious, may have the effect of increasing the already unpopular image of nursing models among sceptical clinicians.

*Models which received a 'medium' response* In the first round of the 'Delphi' the models of King (1968), Orlando (1961), Peplau (1952), Travelbee (1964), Wiedenbach (1964) and Riehl (1974) were only marginally favoured by the respondents. On average these models received five first preference responses each. They tend to describe the 'how of nursing care' rather than what nurses 'do' or 'why' they do it (Meleis, 1985).

Fitzpatrick and Whall (1982) declared that Peplau's work is directly related to psychiatric nursing practice and is readily applicable to the nurse patient situation. Further, Peplau's emphasis on the importance of building interpersonal relationships may be extremely pertinent for the future community placement of these patients. Taking these factors into account it was surprising that it presented little attraction to the respondents. This may be due to two factors: its psychoanalytical undertones - a form of therapy rarely practised on long-stay psychiatric wards in Britain and its American predisposition - a factor already discussed above.

*Models which received a 'weak' or non-response* The work of Levine (1966), Johnson (1959), Rogers (1970), Roy (1971), Fitzpatrick (1983) and Parse (1981) fall into the category of those models that 'describe the why of nursing' (Meleis, 1985). They received, on average, less than one first preference response each. Consistency in respondents' answers was reflected through the fact that Fitzpatrick's (1983) and Parse's work (1981) are directly derived from that of Rogers (1970), a theorist whose conceptualization of nursing may best be described as nonconformist.

A reason for the lack of preference may be found in the preparation many of these nurses received during their initial training. The World Health Organization (1985) stated that in the past nurses were seldom encouraged to ask how or why, rather they were expected to get on with 'doing the job'. Therefore their training and experience with its emphasis on an unquestioning attitude may have had some bearing on their selection of an appropriate model.

In addition, the high untrained to trained staffing ratio (Salvage, 1985) and the low staff to patient ratio (Sutton, 1981) commonly seen on long-stay psychiatric wards may favour a nursing model that concerns itself with getting on with doing the job rather than questioning how or why they do it. As referred to above, many patients in this setting may have to be 'toileted, washed, dressed and fed,' - tasks that need to be done; a questioning attitude towards care strategies may come low in the carers' order of priorities.

Nevertheless, it is possible that coping in the community would be very difficult for patients whose care in hospital was structured around a model that emphasized 'doing' things for patients. The literature reviewed in chapter four shows that extra resources to support such individuals are not always available outside of the large institutions. However, it must be emphasized that models of this type also focus on the promotion of independence and self reliance in human needs and not just 'doing' for others.

*Model choice ('Delphi' round two)*

Those 'model statements' selected by over 51% of the ward managers in the first round of the 'Delphi' were returned to them in the second round. This included the frameworks of Roper et al (1980), Minshull et al (1986) and Henderson (1966). Their anonymity was retained and respondents were asked to rank them into first, second and third preferences depending on how they perceived them as suitable for long-stay psychiatric patient care.

As referred to above, all three models are based on 'Maslow's Hierarchy of Needs'(1954), a theory that is "one of the most influential for nursing models" (Walker and Campbell, 1989 p.56). The HNM of Minshull et al (1986) concentrates less on the physiological needs of the individual and more on the higher psychosocial needs. For example, it has been estimated that devotion to physical aspects of patient care accounts for 57% of Henderson's model, 58% of Roper et al's model, but only 25% of Minshull et al's model (Minshull et al, 1986). This predisposition towards a high element of psychosocial care while recognising the importance of physical care may have influenced the respondents in their choice of model.

The balance of psychosocial and physical care in a simple British nursing model has not gone unnoticed by practitioners. The HNM has recently been chosen for implementation by midwives (Henderson, 1990), by oncology nurses (Kershaw, 1990) and by accident and emergency nurses (Ali, 1990). Furthermore from personal correspondence with one of its originators it is being used in several psychiatric units throughout the United Kingdom (Turner, 1990).

But it could be claimed that models like the HNM help practising nurses to perpetuate the status quo. In contemporary psychiatric nursing we are constantly reminded of the need to innovate and undertake constructive clinical change. This is, without doubt, a valuable quality in any emerging profession and the desire for practitioners to be involved in selecting a nursing model for implementation is a laudable endeavour. However, by asking ward managers to choose a model which is suitable for the care of the long-stay psychiatric patient, one may be accused of preserving current practices. It could be argued that, since fifty one (54%) of the respondents have worked in long-stay areas for six years or more, they were likely to select a model that reflects the care patterns they have always adhered to and which validates, albeit theoretically, their current practice.

Although a valid criticism this accusation must be weighed against the widespread assertions in the literature that ward managers must play the leading role in model selection (Pearson, 1986; Farmer, 1986). After all, they know their patients and are aware of the practical difficulties inherent in their caring environment. The literature suggests that the type of patient (Cowan, 1986) and the type of ward setting (Collister, 1986) should help dictate the nursing model selected. If we accept this, one can ask who else but the ward manager is better qualified to make the selection. Furthermore if by their choice of nursing model the respondents were aiming to preserve the medical model ethos one would have expected them to select more models from the 'systems theory' stable. Results show that this did not happen.

*An eclectic approach to model selection*

When given the opportunity of formulating an eclectic model by selecting elements from various model statements only 27% of the respondents did this. This may contradict Reed (1987), an American mental health nurse, who assumed that most psychiatric nurses take an eclectic approach with nursing models. Of those who did avail themselves of the opportunity, most selected elements from the behavioural models. This supports both the findings from the theoretical bases and the 'model matrix' instruments. The possible reasons why the respondents were attracted to the behavioural models are outlined above.

There is no reason why practitioners cannot use a blend of several nursing models. Figure 5.8 (see p.66) shows that a minority of the respondents use a mixture of Orem (1980) and Roper et al's (1985) work. However practitioners should be aware that models could lose whatever scientific rigour they possess if mixed to form a 'hybrid model'.

*Reasons for respondents' choice of model*

Results show that the type of patients on the ward and the type of ward environment were identified as the most important factors influencing ward managers' choice of model. This reflects the opinions of Griffiths and Christensen (1982) and the Nursing Theories Conference Group (1985) respectively. In addition forty respondents (42%)

80

stated that their selection of a nursing model was determined by their views regarding what they believe long-stay psychiatric nursing was about. This too, has been mentioned in the literature as a valid justification for model selection (Adam, 1985).

There has also been much written concerning the jargon used by nurse theorists in the formulation of their conceptual frameworks. Not only has it been blamed for model implementation difficulties but also for its potential influence on the selection of an appropriate framework (Wright, 1990). It has already been stated that wording/ terminology was mentioned as an influencing factor by only nine respondents (9.5%).

Wright (1988) suggests that models must have flexibility. This property of flexibility was seen by nine respondents (9.5%) as an important selection criterion for their choice of model. It was essential to them that the framework chosen should be compliant enough for easy application to a wide range of day to day patient care situations. Therefore, even the most apposite framework may be self limiting and would require a certain amount of clinical moulding. This is illustrated by the following comments from respondents:

You've got to tailor them to suit the individual patient needs.

Only acceptable to the busy nurse if they can be modified.

It is difficult to understand why there was a significant relationship (although small) between the variables sex and age and choice of model. In his thesis Barker (1988, p.191) states that society typically associates males with reason and rationality and females with irrationality. If these stereotypes are supported one would expect in the present study that the more mechanically minded male respondents would select models with their theoretical basis in systems theory. There is no evidence that this occurred.

*Knowledge concerning nursing models*

While most respondents (91.6%) had been aware of the existence of nursing models, their level of knowledge about them was poor. Together they could remember the names of eight nurse theorists, (Roper, Orem, Henderson, Roy, Riehl, Rogers, Johnson, Peplau), possessing only a limited intimacy with the work of two of these - namely Orem (1980) and Roper et al (1985). It was interesting that only one respondent had heard of Peplau's framework for psychiatric nursing. This illustrates the general unfamiliarity with American nursing models. The exception to this was their awareness of Orem's work, due perhaps to its high profile in Northern Ireland's psychiatric nursing curricula.

81

In comparison, a Canadian study into psychiatric nurses' usage of nursing models by Martin and Kirkpatrick (1987) found that in a 'psychiatric tertiary care facility' the practising nurses were familiar with the models of Peplau, Orlando, Orem, Roy, Nightingale and Rogers. As shown, four of these models are common to both studies. However in contrast to the present study, Kirkpatrick and Martin's respondents were most familiar with Peplau. This partial transatlantic contrariety was not surprising considering the American origins of these models and the concentration of the North American psychiatric nurse training system on nurse-patient psychotherapeutic interventions.

Results of the present study also show that thirty seven of the interviewees (38.9%) stated that they had never read any books or articles relating to conceptual frameworks in nursing. However, it must be remembered that this scenario is not unique to psychiatric nursing nor to Northern Ireland and could be due to the lack of library resources in most of the psychiatric hospitals surveyed. Where a library did exist its opening times rarely coincided with the practising nurses' off duty periods.

Of the ninety five ward managers, thirty (31.6%) claimed that they were using a model of nursing on their ward at the time of interview. This percentage figure was similar to those found in the research by Martin and Kirkpatrick (1987) and Jacobson (1987). These comparatively lower American percentages are surprising considering that models of nursing have been in existence in North America for a greater length of time. Could it be, as Webb (1986) claims, that American nurses are beginning to reject nursing models after many fruitless years of struggling with their implementation? A pertinent question could be is there a probability that a similar repudiation could occur in the United Kingdom. Without educational and management support for model implementation this scenario could indeed occur.

Street (1986) found that what psychiatric nurses say they do in the interview situation and what they actually do when observed may be entirely different. Therefore without having checked their replies with some form of participant or non participant observation (to see if they were using models in practice) the authenticity of these responses must be open to question. Nevertheless, the existence of appropriate documentation was noted but lack of time restricted any effort to investigate whether it was properly used.

Fifty eight respondents (61%) stated that they had received information pertaining to nursing models from nurse management. In the main this took the form of photocopied journal articles distributed directly to the ward by nursing officers or delivered through the internal mail system. These items were normally pinned to the office notice board. Often newly arrived student nurses would be 'told to read them' and it was admitted that 'not all trained staff' did so. According to Chapman (1990) this is not an uncommon finding.

In addition, although twenty six of these respondents (26.5%) stated that they had attended in-service training where nursing models 'were mentioned', ward managers said they had not received any tangible information from nurse educators. This finding may reflect the continued dichotomy that exists between education and practice in the field of psychiatric nursing - a fact highlighted by Cormack (1983). There was an overwhelming concern among respondents that they would not get the required training to help them use nursing models correctly. They had experienced this dearth of information with the nursing process and feared it was being repeated with nursing models. Several respondents made comments such as:

> With the process we were just told to get on with it. As a result we were left helpless. With the current financial stringencies this is bound to happen again with models.

> If staff education on models is good and effective, their implementation should enhance and benefit the overall care of the patient.

When the ward managers were asked to identify the most appropriate method by which clinical staff could be introduced to nursing models, formal lectures and study days came low in their order of preference. The following comments illustrate this point:

> You are sent to study days where there is prolonged note taking from chalkers and talkers - the end result ends up in the ward drawer seldom if ever to be referred to.

Most respondents favoured the use of workshops where participants could get 'hands on' experience using pertinent documentation with hypothetical patients. A substantial number also showed a penchant towards seeing models working in real life situations and talking to those who actually use them. Martin and Kirkpatricks' (1987) respondents had a similar preference.

*Potential problems with model implementation*

Sixty six respondents (69.5%) believed that nursing staff may experience certain problems when trying to implement models of nursing. The main area of concern related to the heterogeneity of patients found in long-stay psychiatric wards. As pointed out above, wards may have many patients with learning difficulties, elderly patients and disturbed patients. How, asked the respondents, were they expected to cater for them all within one model.

*Potential problems with model implementation*

Perhaps a reason for this state of affairs has been identified in the writings of Stevens (1979, p.106). She argues that since patients are grouped on wards for physicians' reasons, nurses are forced to apply nursing models to a given unit population as a secondary rather than as a primary organizational structure. Therefore, because nurses seldom determine the patient population of a ward, these individuals may have widely dissimilar nursing needs - making it difficult for one model to be all-embracing in that setting.

Consequently no nursing model will provide practising nurses with the 'keys to the kingdom'. Even if respondents found an appropriate model it would not cover all eventualities and work in all patient care situations; a view shared by Kristjanson et al (1987). The following comments were indicative of a general feeling among the respondents:

> One model is not enough to cover all the day to day activities of a whole ward full of patients.

> People expect too much from nursing models and I fear they will be let down.

Respondents also identified potential problems in the practical application of nursing models, especially the issue of legalistic documenting; a perception echoed by de la Cuesta's (1979) research into the nursing process. Many of those ward managers surveyed were not trained in the writing skills necessary for the formulation of care plans. To them nursing models were synonymous with endless writing.

> I will reject them if they involve a lot of repetitive writing.

> They encourage the current trend in the unbounded documenting that accompanies litigation anxiety.

This latter problem is not a new one in nursing. Corwin (1961) noted the disparity between clinical reality at ward level and the bureaucratic mechanisms of the hospital. In a minority of cases in the present study there appeared to exist an undercurrent of suspicion regarding the presumed role of nurse administration in the introduction of nursing models. For instance, some of the respondents appeared to view the introduction of nursing models as a management ploy:

Models are going to come in anyway whether we like it or not.

Nursing models are the nursing officer's latest bandwagon the same as patient groupwork and the nursing process once was.

Results also show that some respondents believed that staff-related problems would affect the proper introduction of a nursing model at ward level. Interestingly, only a small minority of these respondents commented that staff numbers should be increased.

We must have the staff resources to implement them or they will fall on 'stony ground'.

A more common concern pertained to the problem of permanent ward staff being moved to cover shortages elsewhere. In most hospitals within the province this unpopular practice was a daily occurrence. Ward managers were often incensed when a 'good nurse', knowledgeable and actively involved in a particular aspect of patient care, was removed to another ward. The following remarks were not uncommon:

We don't need more staff to implement models - we just need to keep the staff we have.

For me to use a model I need staff consistency rather than more staff.

It was realized that the movement of permanent nurses from ward to ward may have been a topical issue at the time of the research. Therefore an interview concerning nursing models could have been an opportunity for them to voice their dissent with this practice.

*Respondents' beliefs regarding the essential elements*

Respondents were asked to identify their personal beliefs about health, nursing, person and the environment from a number of options. These options were obtained from the literature and included as a method of corroborating their model choice from the 'model matrix'.

*Health* Forty four ward managers (46.3%) maintained that health was represented by 'psychological, social and physiological wellbeing', whilst sixteen respondents (16.8%) believed that health was manifestly 'a sense of mental and physical comfort'.

Both these explanations correspond well to behavioural models in general and the HNM in particular. Only four respondents (4.2%) felt that health was 'a positive way of adapting to stresses'. Again this reflects the poor response to systems theory and systems models seen in the 'theoretical bases' and 'model matrix' instruments respectively.

*Nursing* According to sixty nine ward managers (72.6%), nursing was 'a process that helps the patient carry out his/her basic needs so as to promote independence'. Here, too, one can detect the essence of behavioural theory and consequently the behavioural models. In addition, those interpretations of nursing that exemplified systems, developmental, or interactional models were conspicuous by the modicum of support they received. Therefore the results from this section of the interview schedule support the findings from the other two research instruments. Only two respondents (2.1%) believed nursing was 'an intervention to prevent ill health' - thus illustrating an almost total rejection of the old medical model ethos.

*Environment* Some conceptual models of nursing (Levine, 1966; Roy, 1971; Neuman, 1972) take cognizance of an 'internal environment'. As a concept this received little support from respondents. Rather they perceived the environment as an external factor with the largest number, forty seven (49.5%), believing it to be 'an area where man functions'. By putting forward this view they were in complete agreement with the beliefs inherent in the HNM. Again their response helps authenticate the results obtained from the model matrix.

*Person* When respondents were asked what they believed 'the person' was, thirty four (35.8%) choose to indicate that it was 'a unique individual who is constantly learning and changing'. This represents a view supportive of the developmental models. Twenty two (23.2%) claimed the person was 'a whole person who has certain basic needs' and eighteen (18.9%) that he or she was 'a biological, psychological, sociocultural individual'. These latter responses would reflect behavioural models and how the respondents envisaged health and nursing. Therefore the apparent support for developmental models represents a certain conceptual inconsistency among respondents.

Perhaps with their perceptions of health and nursing, respondents were considering 'the patient', whereas here they were asked to consider their views on 'the person'. It is feasible that they differentiated between these two designations, attributing to 'the patient' what Parsons (1952) identified as the 'sick role' while assigning no such dependent status to 'the person'. There is the possibility that if the respondents had been asked what they believed 'the patient' was, a different response would have been obtained.

Apart from these incongruent views regarding 'the person', this section of the interview schedule appears to have been an effective means of checking (and supporting) the findings of the 'model matrix'. However, it could be suggested that the respondent's replies to this section may have been unduly influenced by their previous exposure to the 'model matrix' statements.

*Positive opinions concerning nursing models*

Contemporary psychiatric nursing in Northern Ireland has recently witnessed major changes in the way patients are cared for. Both the new mental health legislation (DHSS NI, 1986) and the 'community shift' have affected grassroot nursing practice. Many comments from the respondents indicate that the introduction of nursing models was important for their professional progression.

> Nursing has changed and we have to keep up to date.

> Nurses need to be kept aware of these things - being in a training ward helps.

In addition theoretical innovations were seen as a possible means of increasing the status of the psychiatric field of nursing care. Some respondents believed that mental nursing was the 'poor relation' compared to general nursing and appeared to envy the perceived prestige of that specialty.

> Nursing models are a new thing. We must keep abreast of them or we will be left behind general nursing.

However, from among those who supported the introduction of nursing models there were others who expressed certain misgivings. For example, thirty five per cent of them feared that even though they may be beneficial, models were just another one of nursing's passing fads.

> I agree they are necessary but I hope it is not going to be a nine day wonder where a lot of effort will eventually be wasted.

> I hope they will not go the same way as team nursing, patient allocation and the nursing process. When I think of all the effort and paperwork that went into those self limiting innovations I cringe!

These opinions have also been echoed in the literature. Wright (1986) and Botha (1989) wonder if models are merely another one of the fashions that nursing indulges in from time to time. If this is the case such passing trends may be detrimental not only to practitioners' confidence in innovative care strategies, but also to the whole fabric of psychiatric nursing.

Other opinions put forward by the ward managers pertained to the practical usefulness of nursing models. In 1984 Greaves argued that nursing models must be tested to establish their validity to real life practice. However, few, if any, of the existing frameworks have undergone any such systematic scientific testing in mental health care. Respondents' responses show that they were aware of this shortcoming and discouraged by the implications of it.

No point in implementing a nursing model if one year later the patient condition hasn't changed.

I would like to see them tested in psychiatric nursing practice.

Opinions were also expressed that perhaps models may help respondents with the proper implementation of the nursing process. It is widely believed in the literature that trying to use the nursing process without the guiding structure of a nursing model is equivalent to 'nursing in the dark' (Aggleton and Chalmers, 1986). Many respondents agreed with this belief and held the expectation that a nursing model would enable them to employ the nursing process correctly, especially in the difficult area of goal setting and evaluation.

They will help us to look at our assessment of patients and the evaluation of care in a different light.

They are useful in their attempt to give guidance to the nurse in the formulation of patient care plans.

Similar results were found in other research. For example, in Martin and Kirkpatrick's (1987) study 97 out of the 107 psychiatric nurses surveyed considered that a nursing model would greatly help them in the application of the nursing process to patient care settings.

*Negative opinions concerning nursing models*

Negative perceptions towards nursing models are not novel. Stevens (1979) noted similar attitudes in the United States and felt that a possible explanation for their occurrence may be due to ...the imposition of intellectually complex concepts upon a discipline previously associated with an anti-intellectual philosophy. (p.213). However, since many innovations in clinical nursing tend to be imposed from above with little regard for the views of busy practitioners (Webb, 1986), there may be good reason for the presence of these attitudes. The heavy-handed imposition of the nursing process in some areas is a case in point and no doubt contributed to the negative opinions concerning nursing models.

Some respondents stated that if a model of nursing was going to be imposed upon them then it had to be an appropriate one.

All models seem to be geared towards general nursing with none catering for psychiatric nursing.

If we're going to spend endless amounts of time, effort, and money getting to grips with a model of nursing I hope to God it will be of benefit to the patients here.

Other respondents, when considering the selection of an appropriate nursing model, appeared not to think of the patients at all. Rather they reflected on whether the chosen model would please intransigent staff.

Certain staff will be awkward about this. It will be difficult to get a suitable model to win them over.

In her research into general nursing, Fretwell (1978) recognized such attitudes as problematic to the smooth transition towards a professional model of care. She identified an in-built desire for routine among some nurses that militated against any form of innovation. She reasoned that these staff were afraid to abandon safe conventions in case they could not cope with the new workload or in case they made mistakes.

There was also the feeling among some respondents that nursing models would interfere with the smooth running of the ward:

A ward manager with suitable staff can organize the care on his ward without any outside interference from nursing models.

If you are a capable nurse you don't need them.

Other respondents pointed out that nursing care has been practised skillfully for years without the encumbrance of explicit nursing models.

We have our own models built over twenty five years - whether the recognized ones are better is highly debatable.

Before models were thought of our practice was every bit as good.

Webb (1986) stressed the ethical problem facing nurses when they identify patient problems for which there is no solution. Many negative comments from respondents in this study contained the word 'idealistic'. They felt that with current resources the delivery of basic psychiatric nursing care was complicated and time consuming enough without encouraging staff to strive for utopian impracticalities. The following remarks were not uncommon among respondents:

Some models have gone over the top and by doing so have lost a great deal of credibility.

We are inclined to chase rainbows and set idealistic and unachievable goals.

These points perennially appear in the literature (Draper, 1990), evidence again that the dichotomy between theory and practice is not diminishing. Nursing models are recognized as concentrating on what 'ought to be'. However, what ought to be is often considered impractical to the ward based nurse who is more interested in 'what is'.

**Limitations**

*The 'theoretical bases' instrument*

Although the results obtained from the 'theoretical bases' instrument appear to be supported by the findings both from the 'model matrix' instrument and the interview schedule, certain aspects of its structural make-up may lead one to question its validity. In essence it was composed of short summaries of the four main theories. Although these were obtained directly from the literature, it may be suggested that the wording used to illustrate behavioural theory was more attractive than, for example, systems theory. The possible effect of wording on decision making has been referred to in the literature review (Tversky and Kahneman, 1981). To counteract this, attempts were made to ensure that each respondent understood the fundamentals of each theory. This was achieved by the consistent use of prepared structured elaborations.

There is also the very real possibility that the theoretical perspective favoured by a particular ward manager may be entirely different to the one with which he or she plans and/or delivers care in the ward situation. For instance, Tissier (1986) maintains that nurses do not plan care on any theoretical basis of nursing practice but on the prevailing psychiatric ideology of the setting in which they work. The aim of this study was not to try to establish what theory currently underpinned the respondents' practice. Rather it was to discover what theory they believed was the most suitable for long-stay psychiatric patient care.

*The 'model matrix'*

For pragmatic purposes, outlines of how each nursing model viewed the 'essential elements' were presented to the research respondents. This strategy has been supported in the literature (Fawcett, 1984). However, when making a choice of a particular model statement respondents were only considering these elements - they were not studying the model in its entirety. It is possible that an inappropriate model may explicate these essential elements in simple terms, while an appropriate model may expound them in indecipherable jargon. Nevertheless Fawcett (1989) argues that these four concepts give the reader a perfect representation of the model in miniature.

Another criticism may be that most nurse managers had very little knowledge and expertise regarding nursing models. This is, according to Chavasse (1987), a very important requirement for proper model selection. However, as McFarlane (1986) states, all nurses have beliefs and values concerning the concepts of nursing, health, person and environment. The respondents were asked to read carefully and select elements that suited their patients and their view of long stay psychiatric patient care. Their lack of erudition concerning nursing models was not seen as an encumbrance in this task.

It must also be borne in mind that in reality it is unrealistic for busy ward managers to be 'au fait' with a wide range of nursing models. If respondents were asked to identify a suitable model of nursing without being shown the 'model matrix', because of their lack of knowledge a minority (8.4%) would have been unable to respond. In addition a majority would have suggested Orem's model or Roper et al's model simply because these theorist's names have been well publicized in the province. Similarly, because none of the research respondents had previously heard of the HNM it would not have been selected at all. Their choice would have been restricted to either those frameworks they had heard of, or those that their managerial or educational colleagues had recommended. Compared to this approach the employment of the 'model matrix' was a more objective and complete stratagem.

Although Aggelton and Chalmers (1986) stress that it is erroneous to choose nursing models by an intuitive act of personal preference, to some extent the 'model matrix' encouraged the respondents to do exactly this. One can ask if, as the literature suggests, ward managers should be the ones to choose a model how else can these individuals do so if they do not have an in-depth knowledge of the area. Silva (1977) argues that intuition based on years of practice is a valuable model selection resource.

The literature also informs us that there are approximately forty nursing models in existence. However, the 'model matrix' only represented nineteen of these. This fact may appear to restrict the amount of choice available to the respondents hence introducing selection bias. The rationale behind the decision to limit the number of models within the 'model matrix' was because some were in the early stages of development and had not been widely published, for example Castledine's systems model (1986). Others were so similar to existing models as to be redundant, for example Kinlein's (1977) model is largely a reproduction of Orem's work. Further most of the models included in the 'model matrix' have been judged by psychiatric nurses as "the most influential in the shaping of nursing knowledge." (Fitzpatrick and Whall, 1983 p.4).

*The interview schedule*

Within the interview schedule there should have been more Likert-type questions. This may ease the testing of reliability. Furthermore, although results that uncover respondents' opinions regarding nursing models are interesting for the research reader, they may be coloured by individual misconceptions. For example, even though the idea of nursing models is a much publicized one it will obviously have a different meaning for different ward managers. Therefore their personal understanding of what a nursing model is may affect their response - believing it to be something quite different from other interviewees. Since the amount and type of education respondents had received regarding nursing models varied remarkably, the possibility of misconceptions is enhanced.

*The involvement of ward managers*

It could be possible that ward sisters/charge nurses were not the right grade of staff to be involved in model selection. Perhaps, if asked, senior nurse managers or nurse tutors would have different preferences. However, it must be recognized that their deficiency in recent ward based experience may cast doubt on their ability to make what they believe is an appropriate choice of a practice model.

Reid (1985), in a Northern Ireland study in general nursing noted that ward managers spent most of their time doing administrative tasks while staff nurses undertook most of the clinical work. If one could hypothetically generalize this finding to psychiatric nursing, perhaps staff nurses would be a more apposite grade to involve in choosing a suitable practice model. It may indeed be the case that they would select an entirely different framework than their ward managers. Nevertheless several studies have identified the ward sister/charge nurse as the most important clinical 'key figure' and 'potential change agent' (Alexander and Orton, 1988). Further, Pearson (1986) strongly emphasizes that they are the most fitting model selectors.

Another possible limitation must be highlighted here. Out of the ninety five ward managers surveyed seven worked on non training wards. When compared with the other respondents there did not appear to be any significant difference in their choice of nursing model, their demographic profile or their opinions towards nursing models. However there may have been subtle yet important differences not detected by the research instruments.

*Reliability and validity*

Due to the absence of research tools for enabling appropriate model choice or for estimating opinions towards nursing models, new research instruments had to be formulated. It was possible to claim face and content validity for the research instruments and internal reliability for some aspects of the interview schedule. However, they have not been completely tested for reliability or with the more scientifically rigorous validity tests.

The 'equivalent test' for reliability requires the simultaneous administration of two different forms of the instrument and was inappropriate because there was no alternative form of the instruments available. However, if the findings of the 'theoretical bases' instrument, the 'model matrix' and the interview schedule are examined as separate research tools and compared, a form of 'equivalent test' emerges. For example, results from the 'model matrix' appeared to support those responses made by respondents in the 'theoretical bases' instrument. Similarly, responses to relevant questions in the interview schedule corroborated well with the various selections made by respondents in both the 'theoretical bases' instrument and the 'model matrix'. Even though this may not establish statistical proof of reliability it does suggest that a considerable level of reliability did exist. Yet it is realized that the possibility of unreliability can never be totally eliminated.

*Generalizability of the research findings*

To some extent this discussion has had a narrow perspective with the findings referring to a particular population of psychiatric ward managers, at a particular time, in a particular location. There is no way of knowing if the same results would have emerged had the research been carried out elsewhere in the United Kingdom. Consequently no attempt has been made to suggest that these results have a wider application to other respondents and settings.

The research instruments developed for this study may be suitable for use in other patient care settings both in psychiatric and general nursing. Based upon experience of their research application it is believed that they are not specialty dependent nor specialty specific. Towell (1975) saw that the caring actions of psychiatric nurses varied quite radically depending on the setting in which they were working. Therefore the use of the 'model matrix' in different mental health specialties may uncover diverse, yet appropriate, nursing model preferences.

# 7 Conclusions, implications and recommendations

## Conclusions

Although the main body of this section will relate to the research questions posed, consequences arising from serendipitous findings will also be included. It is realized that one study is not conclusive. However, from the discussion of the findings, the following conclusions can be drawn.

*Conclusions arising from the research questions*

1.  A majority of psychiatric ward managers in long-stay wards in Northern Ireland believed that behavioural theory was an appropriate conceptual source for their clinical practice.

2.  A majority of ward managers on Northern Ireland's long-stay psychiatric wards believed that the HNM of Minshull et al (1986) was an appropriate nursing model for underpinning their clinical practice.

3.  There was a statistically significant relationship between the respondents' choice of nursing model and their age and gender. However this relationship was not a large one and may have been an artifact of the data rather than 'true'.

4.  There was no statistically significant relationship between respondents' choice of nursing model and, general educational background, nursing qualifications, length of time in psychiatric nursing or length of time working on long-stay wards.

5.    Most respondents held a positive opinion regarding nursing models.

6.    There was no statistically significant relationship between choice of nursing model and any positive and/or negative opinions towards nursing models.

*Conclusions arising from serendipitous findings*

1.    The main criteria respondents used when selecting an appropriate model were the type of patient found within that setting and their beliefs concerning long-stay psychiatric nursing.

2.    The majority of respondents were most familiar with the work of Roper et al (1980) and Orem (1980).

3.    Roper et al (1980), Orem (1980) or a combination of both were claimed to be the main nursing models in use on long-stay psychiatric wards in Northern Ireland at the time of the study.

4.    Many respondents had not received any information regarding models of nursing. Of those who did, it mostly took the form of photocopied journal material delivered to the ward.

5.    Other than a few planned study days, nurse educators had given no information or guidance to the respondents on nursing models.

6.    Most respondents anticipated problems with the implementation of nursing models at ward level. They envisaged the greatest potential source of complication as relating to the diversity of patients in such settings.

7.    If given the option, respondents preferred to learn about nursing models in an experiential manner rather than by more formal lecturing methods.

The conclusions indicate that the purposes of part one of the study have been met.

**Implications**

Based on the preceding discussion and conclusions the following implications for nursing practice, administration, education and theory development seem justified. These four areas are interlinked - if one fails to play its proper role the use of nursing models at patient care level could be threatened. However, because the complete reliability and therefore validity of the research instruments has not been statistically demonstrated, such implications may be open to question.

*Implications for practising nurses*

The results show that a behavioural theoretical perspective was an appropriate way of conceptualising the philosophy of care on long-stay psychiatric wards in Northern Ireland. This would suggest that ward based nurses who work in this setting should focus on the basic human needs of their patients be they biological, social or psychological.

The assessment of a patient's care requirements and how care is planned, implemented and evaluated is determined by the particular nursing model being used. It appears from round one of the 'Delphi' that any of those nursing models dealing with independence in human needs could be used on long-stay psychiatric wards. However, according to the results of round two, the HNM was seen by the ward managers as being the most suitable.

The results also indicate that the 'Self Care' model of Orem (1980) was not perceived by the respondents as an appropriate framework for practice. This reflects views from the literature (Collister, 1986; Smith, 1986). Considering that 'Orem' has been strongly recommended for implementation within this setting such a finding has important implications for patients and practitioners alike. It is suggested that practising nurses should be cautious in their adoption of this model.

A majority of respondents rejected most of the American nursing models, preferring instead those that were British in origin. Consequently, perhaps ward based nurses should use only those nursing models that they believe are appropriate to their particular political, economic and health care setting.

Many research reports point to the ward sister as the key agent of change in the clinical area. Practitioners should be aware of this role and use it not as a vetoing strategy for all innovations but as a central component for selecting a relevant model to help improve the quality of patient care. The present study illustrates that, given appropriate methods, clinical nurses were able to choose a nursing model that they believed was suitable not only to their patients but to themselves and the clinical setting in which they practise.

*Implications for nurse educators*

According to Littlewood (1989) and Sullivan (1989) nurse education still takes place within a biomedical framework. This lack of concentration on nursing models by nurse educators was reflected in the results of the present study. Although a small minority had "heard nursing models mentioned at study days", all the ward managers said they had received no information from teaching staff on this topic. Most of the respondents realized the need for change and were positive towards the idea of a more theoretical orientation. However this is not enough, they cannot work in isolation; assistance must be forthcoming from colleges of nursing through intensive continuing education in line with the UKCC (1991) recommendations for Post-registration Education and Practice.

The findings also have implications for what is taught to student nurses. The dichotomy between ward and classroom has been well publicized. If however, prior to placement in long-stay psychiatric areas students were familiar with nursing models in general and the HNM in particular and if experienced ward staff also received this instruction, the ward - classroom divide may be bridged.

Respondents also identified what they believed to be the best methods for teaching qualified nurses about nursing models. Lectures were seen to be of limited use and should be kept to a minimum. Rather, workshops should be organized where participants can get 'hands on' experience with model based practice. The use of hypothetical patients would also ensure that experience could be gained without fear of making a mistake. In addition, staff should be able to see the model in action within similar settings and be able to discuss its advantages and disadvantages with those who use it.

*Implications for managers*

As far as nursing models are concerned, it appears that many long-stay psychiatric wards in Northern Ireland are forgotten and isolated. An indication of the extent of the problem was illustrated by the assertions of thirty seven percent of respondents that they had received no information from nurse management on nursing models, while most respondents complained of a lack of support and guidance from that quarter. This highlights a dearth of communication down the nursing hierarchy regarding an issue that has potentially important implications for patient care. Managers should work in partnership with practitioners, educators and researchers in order to assure open communication on nursing models at every level of the organization.

In the past the nursing process was imposed on ward based nurses and patients; more recently there have been attempts at introducing nursing models in a similar fashion. This is a recipe for widespread theoretical insolvency at patient care level. The avoidance of this scenario can only come about if clinical nursing personnel are involved in selecting the model for practice. If this is carried out correctly, the resultant framework will be acceptable to practitioners and, therefore will possess clinical credibility.

As alluded to above the ward manager has a major role in accepting or rejecting change. After all, it is he or she who controls the ward environment and the norms of care within that environment. From what some respondents said senior nurse managers are naive if they believe that nursing models can be selected and properly introduced without the collaboration of ward sisters/charge nurses. If this is attempted models may be assimilated on paper, but at weekends, evenings or on night duty, nurses may resort to traditional routines and rituals.

The respondents also identified impediments to the successful introduction of nursing models. For example, the high numbers of untrained staff on their wards and the incessant movement of the few trained staff to fill vacancies elsewhere. These factors merit in-depth consideration by managers. They should address the following question: if nursing models are difficult enough to implement in those areas where there are high levels of staff, why penalize poorly staffed areas?

The varied patient mix on a typical long-stay psychiatric ward was also identified as a potential barrier to effective model implementation. This is often the result of patients being allocated to wards by medical diagnosis rather than by their nursing problems. Since the main input in long-stay psychiatric areas is nursing - should not senior managers work towards the distribution of these patients by nursing problem rather than by psychiatric diagnosis?

*Implications for nurse theorists*

In 1972, Altschul found it impossible to obtain any indication of an ideology among psychiatric nurses. From the results of the present study it appears that contemporary practitioners are beginning to realize the importance of using nursing models as a basis for their practice. Further, they were able and willing to put forward their own implicit conceptual values.

Other than Stockwell (1985), nurse theorists on this side of the Atlantic have showed little interest in developing a nursing model for psychiatric practice. This is unfortunate considering the respondents' assertion that models of this type were urgently required. At present ward staff are struggling with little success to mould physically oriented models around the unique area of psychiatric nursing care. The HNM has been chosen as suitable - but perhaps it was selected as the 'best of a bad bunch'.

If British models for psychiatric nursing are to be developed they would need to be versatile enough to cope with the multifarious situations that arise on any ward. Although this may be a utopian brief, it is more realistic than believing that in the future the practising psychiatric nurse will have a repertoire of twenty or thirty nursing models and be able to select different ones depending on which type of patient problems he or she encounters.

## Recommendations

Recommendations will be presented that relate to the limits of the study and possible future directions for nursing research. It is hoped that by giving prominence to certain methodological reconsiderations (discerned by hindsight) other researchers will be imbued with the ideas and motivation to become involved in the present investigator's area of interest.

### Possible replication of the study

It is strongly recommended that the present study is replicated with the following suggested methodological modifications:

If a more extensive and representative pilot study was undertaken it would be possible to exclude those model statements that the pilot group believed were unsuitable for inclusion in the main study. Hence the respondents would be able to make a choice from fewer model statements.

In the second round of the present study the researcher returned to the respondents those model statements favoured by over fifty one per cent of the interviewees in the first round. Although this was a legitimate stratagem, it would be interesting to observe if an individualized return of the first round responses produced a different result.

Furthermore, although ninety five respondents out of a possible ninety eight was a laudable response rate, this relatively small number can result in empty contingency table cells, hence affecting the relationship testing Chi square statistic. Therefore it is recommended that a replication of this work should take place elsewhere on a larger scale.

From Towell's (1975) findings of the differences across psychiatric nursing specialties it is possible that ward managers from diverse areas of psychiatry would select a different nursing model than that chosen by those on long-stay wards.

Consequently to discover whether the findings have a wider application it would be valuable to administer the same instruments in another clinical setting.

*Future research recommendations*

There are several research questions that could form the basis for future investigations. These include:

1.   Does in service education influence the implementation of nursing models?

2.   Has the use of nursing models at ward level had any effect on patient satisfaction?

3.   Has the use of nursing models at ward level had any effect on the job satisfaction of nursing staff?

4.   Has the use of nursing models at ward level had any effect on the atmosphere of the ward?

5.   How are nurses' use of conceptual models viewed by other paramedical disciplines?

6.   Is it more appropriate to employ one nursing model or multiple models on psychiatric wards?

7.   Do those clinical nurses who say they use a recognized nursing model for their practice actually do so?

8.   Would nurse managers and nurse educators (who may be involved in imposing a framework) select the same model for practice as ward based nurses?

9.   What are the reasons why nursing models are undergoing a period of unpopularity in certain areas of the United States? (see Webb, 1984)

10.   What nursing models would patients select as suitable for their care?

11.   Would rigorous testing indicate high levels of reliability and validity for the research instruments used in this part of the study?

**Part one of this study as a foundation for part two**

At the outset it was stressed that part one of this study was a descriptive/exploratory investigation into the selection of an appropriate nursing model by clinical nurse managers. An alternative approach of a more in-depth research project was rejected mainly due to lack of available research based information in this area. However it is suggested that the descriptive/exploratory nature of this part of the study has paved the way for a more penetrating investigation in the second part.

# Part 2
## EVALUATING THE SELECTED NURSING MODEL

# 8 Introduction to part two

## Background

In the first part of this study ward managers were asked to select a nursing model appropriate for their particular patient care requirements. Most of these clinical managers (61%) selected the Human Needs model (HNM) of Minshull et al (1986). For part two it is proposed to facilitate the implementation of the HNM and to evaluate the effect of its use on specific quality of care indicators. Fawcett (1989) refers to this as 'credibility determination'. She states that 'credibility determination' is necessary to avoid the uncritical acceptance of a nursing model and to establish the effect of using a nursing model on the outcomes of nursing care.

In the mid 1980s nursing models were very popular in the British nursing press and practising psychiatric nurses were being encouraged to use them by educators and managers alike. However, it was not immediately apparent what effect their implementation was going to have on the delivery and outcomes of nursing care. One could ask if nursing models were as advantageous as reputed why were most nurses experiencing problems with their implementation; and why were some practitioners so negative towards them.

In 1986 when the research was at an embryonic stage a decision was made to concentrate solely on the area of nursing model selection. However this decision had ethical implications: what would happen if an appropriate model was selected? It did not seem fair to the respondents involved in the study to report these findings and do little else. Furthermore, results from part one showed that respondents stressed the need for models to be 'tried and tested' in psychiatric nursing practice. This was seen as an essential prerequisite before they could be implemented on a larger scale. Therefore part two of the study was an obvious progression from part one.

*Purposes of the second part of the study*

1.  To evaluate how specific structural aspects of care on a long-stay psychiatric ward are affected by the implementation of a selected nursing model.

2.  To evaluate how specific processes of care on a long-stay psychiatric ward are affected by the implementation of a selected nursing model.

3.  To evaluate how specific outcomes of care on a long-stay psychiatric ward are affected by the implementation of a selected nursing model.

*Need for the second part of the study*

Nursing models have been applied, often without question, to a wide range of patient care settings. They have also been seen by various authors as a panacea for problems in nursing practice, education, management and research. This endorsement has been reinforced by the UKCC which has voiced its support for the widespread implementation of nursing models on nurse training wards. Further, several British authors have argued that the introduction of these models into practice was a most important innovation (Pearson, 1986; Castledine, 1986).

However some nurses were worried at what appeared to be unsubstantiated acceptance and support. In the United Kingdom, for instance, nurses like McFarlane (1986) advocated that all nursing models require careful analysis and evaluation in practice. Yet five years later a review of the literature reveals that such empirical information is still not available. As a result, there is little research evidence pertaining to their application, let alone their evaluation.

In the 1980s various government reports stressed the importance of nurses being actively involved in quality assurance. The issues of consumerism, standard setting, quality control, continuous quality improvement and total quality management were widely discussed in nursing journals. Respected nurses wrote that the application of nursing models to patient care would help improve the quality of the service delivered (McFarlane, 1977; Hardy, 1982; Farmer, 1986). Further, results from part one of this present study indicate that many respondents also firmly believed that nursing models would improve the quality of care. However to date no available research report has confirmed the link between the use of a nursing model and the quality of care delivered to, or received by, patients.

Therefore, using Lippitt's (1973) theory of change the second part of this study focuses on evaluating the effects nursing models have on certain specified resources of care (Structure), nursing actions (Process) and the end results of care (Outcomes).

## The human needs model (HNM)

Because this study involves the use of the HNM a brief introduction to the model is necessary. A more detailed account of the HNM can be found in Minshull et al (1986).

In 1986 Minshull and colleagues from a Manchester school of nursing wanted to formulate a nursing model that suited British culture, nurse education and health care system. Their central tenet was that it had to be understandable to all levels of nursing staff and easily translated into practice.

As tutors Minshull and her colleagues knew that most nurses were already familiar with Maslow's (1954) different levels of human need. They decided to use his work as the theoretical foundation for their Human Needs Model (HNM). Maslow's theory has been used to underpin other models (Henderson, 1966; Roper et al, 1980; Orem, 1980) and has been used as a category for classifying models by Meleis (1985). Maslow identified five basic human needs: Physical, Safety, Affiliation, Esteem and Self Actualization. Within the HNM each patient is a unique individual different from all others and in possession of intrinsic value. Some of the human needs may be unmet and the patient may be aware or unaware of the unmet need.

*Physical needs*

According to Minshull et al (1986) individuals must maintain a balance between physical wellbeing and physical illness. This balance must consider the need for: nutrition, elimination, temperature control, mobility, sleep/rest, light/darkness, quietness/noise, oxygen and sensory stimulation. They stressed that an unmet physical need may be life-threatening if ignored. Examples of unmet physical needs include airway obstruction, dehydration and hunger.

*Safety and security needs*

The philosophy behind the HNM maintains that people require a safe, orderly, organized and predictable life. Long stay psychiatric patients need a certain amount of routine, financial and social stability and familiar and stable surroundings. These patients need to feel safe and secure. Unmet needs in this category may result in anxiety, disorientation, abnormal behaviour and physical danger.

*Affiliation needs*

These is a strong need for people to have contact, to belong and to be accepted by others. Although some psychiatric patients like solitude, most need positive relationships with other people such as fellow patients, family, staff, friends or relatives. Unmet needs here result in loneliness, friendlessness, rejection, rootlessness and alienation.

*Dignity and self esteem needs*

All human beings require a level of positive self esteem. Patients want privacy sometimes, the respect of others, to be involved in decision making, to be appreciated, to get recognition, to have their dignity respected. Here unmet needs result in dependence, loss of self respect, loss of motivation and degradation.

*Self actualization needs*

The HNM specifies that all people need the opportunity to be individualistic and to achieve their full potential. Although not everyone will reach this level, everyone should be allowed to strive for it if they wish. At this level of need individuals can explore new areas of interest and perhaps achieve new potential.

*The life continuum*

The HNM sees the person on a line between:

| MAXIMAL | | MAXIMAL |
|---------|---|---------|
| WELLNESS | ———————— | ILLNESS |
| (Independence) | | (Dependence) |

The nurse may determine a patient's position on this continuum objectively by signs, clinical features, conversation and behaviours. Patients may also offer subjective information based on their thoughts and feelings.

Since nurses in long-stay psychiatric wards may be caring for some patients who are relatively well, their role within this model is a supportive one. Support may be given either directly or indirectly to enable the patient to proceed towards maximal wellness and independence. The nature of the support required by patients will depend on their need for nursing.

The HNM uses a four stage nursing process for its implementation. The nurse, with the assistance of the patient and others, assesses how the patient functions in each of the five levels of need. From this collaborative appraisal, actual and potential problems are identified. This is followed by the setting of mutual goals that are realistic and achievable. With the assistance of the patient, his or her family and other professionals, interventions are planned and carried out. The results of these interventions are evaluated to see how far the set goals have been achieved.

In summary, the HNM is constructed on the assumption that everyone has five levels of human need that are important for living. People with mental health problems may have unmet needs at any of these levels. Through the use of a collaborative nursing process these unmet needs will be identified and attempts will be made to fulfil them.

# 9 Literature review: using nursing models

**Issues concerning the application of nursing models**

In the present literature review it is proposed to focus on those issues that affect the use of nursing models in practice. These include:

the relationship between nursing models and practice;
the theory-practice gap;
relevant issues in the application of models in practice;
research into the testing and application of nursing models;
research into the effects of nursing models in practice;
the affects of nursing models on quality of care;
methods of organising nursing work.

*The relationship between nursing models and practice*

Clark (1982) wrote that nursing practice without models was like someone going to sea without a map in a ship without a rudder. The uniqueness of this theoretical relationship had been specified much earlier by Dickoff and James (1968). They stated that theory is born in practice, is refined in research and must and can return to practice. Lerheim (1991) uses the analogy of a coin to explain the relationship: one side is nursing knowledge with its abstract concepts, models and theories; the other side is nursing practice. She stresses that, like a coin, theory and practice is a unity and must be seen as a whole.

There are many acclaimed definitions for nursing models that highlight the theory-practice association:

A model for nursing practice is a systematically constructed, scientifically based, and logically related set of concepts which identify the essential components of nursing practice together with the theoretical bases for these concepts and the values required in their use by the practitioner.

(Riehl and Roy, 1974, p.3).

Models are essential tools for guiding practice and or making the values, assumptions and goals of our practice explicit.

(McFarlane, 1986, p.115).

Other writers acknowledge that the link between models and practice is necessary for nursing's claim to be a profession. For instance, Chalmers (1989) argues that without a strong relationship between the work of nurse theorists and the work of practitioners the basic requirement of a profession is missing. Botha (1989) supports this view asserting that only if nursing is able to prove that this link exists will it be a 'legitimate contender' for professional status.

Fawcett (1989) specified three criteria by which the worth of a nursing model can be appraised. These are:

Social utility - Does the model include explicit rules for practice?

Social significance - Does the model lead to nursing actions that make important differences for the patient?

Social Congruence - Does the model lead to nursing activities that meet the expectations of society? (p.51).

These criteria highlight the importance of the idea that clinical practice and nursing models should have a reciprocal relationship. However, this idea is open to challenges. Smoyak (1988), an American psychiatric nurse theorist, points out that some models are not intended to be clinically relevant. Referring to Martha Rogers's nursing model (1970) Smoyak suggests that it is not meant for application in practice and that it never was. She quotes Rogers herself as saying that her model is a stimulus for thinking and that it may even be dangerous to apply it directly to practice.

Those who agree that models are not necessarily tools for practice do so from the following philosophical stance: models are by their very nature abstract and so they originate from and lead to abstract thinking. That is part of their value. Since many

111

are at the forefront of new knowledge development they are extending nursing's scientific frontiers. Therefore by definition, they cannot coincide with what is now being practised. Moreover, to make all models clinically relevant would hamper the development of more abstract ideas that might eventually prove more valuable to nursing.

Those who favour the opposing point of view take the following philosophical stance: regardless of whether nurses work as researchers, educators, theorists, administrators or practitioners it must be realized that nursing is a practice profession with the patient at the receiving end of that practice. Therefore nursing models should have a direct bearing on patient care. If they do not, their value is open to question.

So it can be argued that there are two types of nursing models available to the profession: the 'realistic' that coincides with the views of practitioners and the 'idealistic' that may appear alien to contemporary practitioners. Draper (1991) believes that an overemphasis on the importance of the latter group has retarded British nurses' understanding of the real world of practice. It is obvious that the selected HNM belongs to the former group.

*The theory practice gap*

There have been several research studies that have highlighted the existence of a 'theory-practice gap' (Bendall, 1975; Nolan, 1989). This commonly refers to the dichotomy that exists between what students are taught in colleges of nursing and what they experience in clinical practice. The resultant frustration, stress and disillusionment may be more acute in the examination situation. In his thesis on psychiatric nurse education in Britain, Clinton (1981) pointed out that if students wrote down in a nursing examination what they practised in reality they would fail. In 1991, Merchant noted that the theory-practice gap was still a problem for many nursing students.

However, the divide between theory and practice does not just affect nursing students. It may be apparent to qualified staff that their methods of assessing, planning, implementing and evaluating care bear little resemblance to what the journal articles or textbooks suggest. This may cause them to experience cognitive dissonance. Festinger (1964) used this term to explain the anxiety experienced by those whose behaviour is inconsistent with their values. If nurses accept the theoretical basis of nursing as part of their value system, then they may experience cognitive dissonance when they find that these values are inconsistent with what they practise. Similarly, while examining possible reasons why nurses left the profession, Kramer (1974) used the term 'reality shock' to explain the phenomenon that occurs when practitioners cannot cope with the obvious divorce between theory and practice.

But what effect do nursing models have on the theory-practice gap? Perhaps rather than bringing practice and principles closer together nursing models are doing the opposite. Biley (1991) would concur with this, pointing out that nursing is still entrenched in traditional methods of caring and the introduction of nursing models creates confusion and hostility hence perpetuating the gap.

There is consensus in the literature that models should emerge from practice and return to practice. However in reality models of nursing invariably come from an academic background and as Jones (1990) states "theorists have been away from practice and the reality of nursing for many years." (p.22).

Therefore, since most models are not being formulated by practising nurses, this encourages the theory-practice gap to remain. Wright (1988) explained that:

Nursing models can make nursing more remote from practice: esoteric notions which keep the ivory tower nurse happy but which fail to reach down to the coalface of reality. (p.154).

In taking a broader view Meleis (1985) felt that:

Nurse theorists were developing theories in isolation, researchers pursued questions of interest only to educators and administrators and practitioners pursued their practices whilst oblivious to what the other two groups were doing. (p.50).

Although Meleis writes in the past tense there is little evidence to suggest that the situation has changed.

There are other possible reasons why nursing models may lead to a widening of the theory-practice gap. Some of these have already been discussed in part one of this study. They include the American origin of various nursing models and the jargon used by nurse theorists to structure their models. According to Jones (1989) much of the division stems from nurse practitioners seeing themselves as 'doers' and the theorists as 'thinkers'.

It is not clear whether nurses would still hold these opinions if they had a better understanding of the models in question. After all many nurses have not been given the time, the opportunity, the support or the education to comprehend them or implement them properly. Furthermore, the perceived contribution of nursing models to the theory-practice gap may have been less if they had not been introduced by nurse management using a 'power-coercive' approach. Lerheim (1991) is not surprised that progress has been slow. She suggests that this is because it takes time for models to pass through various filters and sources to reach practice.

Notwithstanding the views of the above authors there are others who are convinced that it is only by using nursing models that theory and practice may eventually meet (Craig, 1980; Smith, 1986). One way for models to reduce the theory-practice gap is for educators to underpin curricula with nursing models that match practice. If a nursing curriculum is structured around a particular nursing model and the same model is used by practitioners then the theory-practice gap could be bridged for both students and staff. Gould (1989) agrees, warning that if staff on a ward reach consensus on a nursing model that is not known or taught by the college staff - the situation will continue where learners are exposed to one set of ideals in the classroom and another in the clinical areas.

It has been pointed out elsewhere in this thesis that nursing models deal with what 'ought to be' not 'what is'. This poses a dilemma for practising nurses who are more concerned with the 'is' of care. Stevens (1979) argues that like other professions nurses would be better off to start with a clear picture of what is; only then could they progress and set future directions. There is however an important counter argument to this strategy. If nursing models are used that reflect where practice is rather than where it ought to be, nursing may remain entrenched in ritualistic subservience to the medical model.

Nonetheless, Stevens is suggesting that nurses can only feel comfortable with a realistic model that reflects the actuality of their practice. If faced with introducing an idealistic and conceptually foreign framework they could succumb to 'reality shock'. Robinson (1990) supports this conclusion stating that the perpetuation of the theory-practice gap can be halted by getting compatibility between the formal nursing model and the practitioners' informal nursing model. Therefore by implementing a model selected by practitioners this study is attempting to bridge the theory-practice gap. Biley (1991) believes that such an endeavour "...can only lead to an improvement in the quality of nursing care." (p.30)

*Relevant issues in the application of models to practice*

*Are models being used in practice?* In part one of this study only thirty two percent of respondents admitted using a nursing model. Other psychiatric nurse researchers found that only twenty two percent of their 64 respondents consistently used a nursing model (Martin and Kirkpatrick, 1987). Although scant attention has been paid to explaining this 'poor uptake', American writers (Meleis, 1985; Kemp, 1990) argue that the reason is simple - nursing models are being applied mainly as guides for education rather than practice. It was only in the mid 1980s that British nurses became interested in nursing models. As in the United States the impetus behind this trend originated mainly with nurse education and administration rather than with practitioners themselves.

In the United Kingdom, Barber (1986) showed his enthusiasm for nursing models, stating that the professional climate of psychiatric nursing was alive to them. But his enthusiasm is not surprising considering that in 1986 most interested nurses were exuberant about nursing models. In that year many British books on nursing models were published and conferences were held throughout Britain to expound the merits of using nursing models.

However in the 1990s nursing models are undergoing more scrutiny and criticism. For instance when referring to their application in practice Melia (1990) said "The only saving grace is that patient care has remained untouched by the dead hand of the model on nursing's tiller. (p.38). It must be remembered that Melia was concluding her contribution to a debate on nursing models. Therefore it is not known if this opinion is genuine or merely reflects her role in supporting or rejecting a particular debating motion. Nevertheless Salvage (1990) stressed that:

> Nurses should not be made to feel guilty if their practice is not based on an explicit model, nor should it be assumed that all progressive practitioners are using one. (p.1).

*How are nursing models being applied?* The literature has many published examples of nursing models being applied to practice. Recently there have been several British publications that employed a care study format to illustrate the use of nursing models (Webb, 1986; Collister, 1988, Chalmers, 1988; Barber, 1990; Easterbrook, 1988; While, 1989). The relative ease of application experienced by most of these authors is contrary to other reports on the use of nursing models. In America Engstrom (1984) saw that practising nurses were becoming frustrated when they tried to use nursing models. Earlier Judson (1980) noted that nursing models made practitioners:

> ...acutely uncomfortable. Their descriptions don't seem to fit what goes on in the doing...they seem too abstract and too limited... and don't prepare one for the variety of things to think about, the variety of obstacles and traps to understanding, the variety of approaches to solution.
>
> (cited in Hardy 1982 p.447).

Such models have to undergo modification to suit the vagaries of particular clinical situations. If this is not done and the model is applied in a rigid fashion, the result may be confusion and apathy. McFarlane (1986) stated that "a model is not a straitjacket - it is a tool which can be adapted for the needs of the job." (p.2). However we should be wary of making radical adaptations to a model less its original theoretical meaning is lost.

*What problems arise when using nursing models?* Because of their broad focus nursing models may equate with Merton's (1968) 'grand theory' categorization and because of this they may have limited value to the practising nurse faced with specific clinical problems. In other words they may be so theoretically broad that they are almost useless. Pearson (1986) identified another problem. He stated that "Real nurses nursing real patients are busy, tired and therefore unable to engage in elaborate conceptual exercises throughout the working day." (p.53). Perhaps many of the perceived problems associated with using nursing models are attitudinal in origin and relate to those negative opinions reported in part one of this study.

*Should practitioners use one model or more than one?* Riehl and Roy (1974) advocated a single model of nursing because such a theoretical approach would unify and lend stability to the profession. However, in later editions of their book (1980) they appeared to favour a multiple model approach. The reason for this turnabout is not explained. However the realization that nursing is becoming increasingly diversified and specialized and that no single model would be adequate to cover all nursing care situations may be a possible explanation.

Kristensen et al (1987) state that the use of only one nursing model in a clinical area forces the practitioner to close prematurely their perception and attend only to those things that the model covers. Therefore it could be argued that theoretical pluralism brings a richness to nursing.

However the use of more than one model can lead to practical managerial problems and these have been referred to in part one of this study (see p.29). Because of these problems there are many who favour a single model approach. Moore (1986) states that if general enough one nursing model can provide guidelines within which to practice (cited in Salvage 1986). Chalmers (1988) said "It is likely that a chosen model can be used in a particular unit for the majority of people cared for there...individuality can be taken too far." (p.3). However, with the large number of models now available the possibility of nursing ever becoming a single model profession is a remote one.

*Nursing models and the nursing process* For more than a decade now nurses in the United Kingdom have been interested in learning about and applying the nursing process (Crow, 1977). The nursing process has at least four designated stages; assessment, planning, implementation and evaluation. In her thesis Cooper (1988) states that these stages represent the logical steps in a problem solving exercise. Therefore all health care professionals use this four stage process. This begs the question what makes the process a nursing process rather than an occupational therapy process or a medical process. The answer is that it depends on the model that is being used. The Nursing Process Evaluation Working Group (1986) pointed out that nurses in the U.K. recognize the need to have a model that guides care planning and provides the rationale for assessment and action coherence.

According to Cooper (1988) "Planning patient care by the use of the nursing process assumes an explicit or implicit model of nursing...." (p.23). Wright (1986) argues that United Kingdom nurses were introduced to the nursing process before they heard about nursing models. He blames this "getting the cart before the horse" for the many problems encountered by nurses in the past when they attempted to apply the nursing process. However it is noteworthy that the application problems have not disappeared now that nurses have gotten both.

Aggelton and Chalmers (1986) believe that using the nursing process without a nursing model is 'nursing in the dark'. They argue that the four stages of the nursing process will not tell a practitioner the who, when, why or what of assessing, planning, implementing and evaluating. A nursing model should provide this guidance. Therefore the nursing process is how nursing models are put into action.

In America Fawcett (1990) wrote "A fully developed conceptual model of nursing...tells the clinician what to assess and how to plan interventions in a general manner and provides global criteria for evaluation." (p.256). This echoes the recent view of writers in the United Kingdom (Walsh, 1990; Crouch, 1990).

However in reality most models of nursing are used in clinical practice as assessment tools only. Webb (1986) points out that they are very useful in giving nurses "...fuller and richer details about their patients." (p.210). Nonetheless, she found when reading care plans that "once the assessment is carried out the model gets lost in the later stages of the nursing process." (p.210).

Luker (1988) disagrees, maintaining that many nurses use models to highlight broad outcomes. However, she does concede that they tend to rely on their existing repertoire of interventions. In a letter to a professional journal Sternberg (1986) maintained that "nursing models may help me write a care plan but they will not change the way I nurse on the ward." (p.12).

Despite these comments models do offer broad guidelines for nursing intervention. For example Roper et al (1983) suggest that the nurse seeks to prevent, solve, alleviate or teach the patient to cope with problems with the activities of living. Orem's self care model (1980) suggests that the nurse uses three nursing systems to do for, support, create a better environment or teach to encourage self care. Therefore perhaps nursing models are not at fault; they are merely the tools. The problems lie with the way that nurses are trying to apply them to patient care.

*Research into the testing of nursing models*

There has been a great deal written about the necessity to test nursing models to provide evidence of the validity and accuracy of their concepts and assumptions (Chinn and Jacobs, 1983). However little progress has been made towards this goal either by the theorists themselves, researchers, or by those nurses who use them in practice. Dickoff and James (1968) recommended such testing claiming that not to do so would have consequences for the quality of care. This is understandable considering the implications of nurses using a model of dubious validity as an organising framework for the care of patients. However in the literature reviewed, what is meant by 'testing' is not made clear nor are authors in agreement on how it should be undertaken.

Following a comprehensive search of the American literature from 1952 to 1985, Silva (1986) found that the use of research to test models was rare; she said that "this is an aspect of science that has remained outside the nursing research mainstream." (p.1).

Using rigid selection criteria Silva located sixty two research studies using the work of one or more of five theorists; Roy, Orem, Newman, Rogers and Johnson. She categorized the studies into three groups:

*Minimal use* In these studies the model was used as a framework for the research but was not integrated further into the study. Twenty four of the sixty two studies reviewed were in this category.

*Insufficient use* In these studies the model was only used to organize the research instruments. Twenty nine of the sixty two studies reviewed were in this category.

*Adequate use* In these studies the researchers meet the following criteria:

1. The research is to determine the validity of a model's assumptions/prepositions.
2. The model is an explicit framework for the research.
3. The relationship between the model and the study's hypotheses is clear.
4. The research hypotheses are deduced clearly from the model's assumptions.
5. The research hypotheses are tested in an appropriate manner.
6. The research provides indirect evidence as to the validity of the model's assumptions/prepositions.
7. The evidence is discussed in terms of how it supports, refutes or explains the model.

Silva identified only nine studies in this category, several of which she felt tested only a part of the model. She concluded that:

> Many studies have used models as frameworks for research but only a few have explicitly tested these models in the sense of trying to determine the underlying validity of the model's assumptions or propositions. (p.8).

Other American 'theory watchers' who have undertaken similar literature searches to that of Silva have come up with comparable findings. In reviewing the journal 'Nursing Research' for the years 1974 to 1985, Beck (1985) noted that only a 'few' research studies involved the testing of nursing models. In 1989 Allen and Hayes undertook a similar project. They found that little had changed in the four years since Silva's work.

In 1990 British nurses like Girot, Burnard and Melia called for the major components within nursing models to be tested. If this call is ignored they felt that models would be seen as the mere speculation of 'armchair theorists'. Earlier Webb (1984) had stated "What these frameworks amount to is no more than a collection of unverified assumptions which reflect the personal philosophies of or value systems of their authors...." (p.22).

Whitehead (1933) in 'The Aims of Education' maintained that any science goes through three stages of development:

1. The stage of romance - ideas are explored and discussed in a fairly cavalier fashion.
2. Stage of precision - ideas are tested rigorously.
3. Stage of generalization - general statements about the discipline can be made because of preceding research.

In referring to Whitehead, Burnard (1990) states that nursing is 'stuck' at the stage of romance.

However, it could be argued that because of their conceptual structure nursing models cannot be tested. Kristenjansen et al (1987) stress that models do not provide the level of specificity required to derive and test principles. Fawcett (1990) agrees, asserting that because the propositions of a nursing model are so abstract and general and the concepts are not operationally defined they are not amenable to testing. There is also the belief that since many models are more philosophic than scientific the lack of empirical testing is justified (Uys, 1987).

Chapman (1990) endorses these views. He bases his endorsement on Kuhn's assertion (1970) that models are valuable not as testable theories but as a preparadigm stage of scientific development. As such they are broad abstract frameworks describing relationships between concepts from which can emerge testable hypotheses. But there is little evidence of any such emergence. Green (1985) believes that the vague non-specific terms used in many nursing models are hardly likely to lead to testable hypotheses.

Therefore one would suspect that it should be a cause for concern that untested models are being used as a basis for patient care and for the education of nurses? Green (1988) appears to disagree explaining that:

> There is a genuine need for applicable nursing models and...these are useful even if unsupported by scientific research, as long as no claims are made for more supporting evidence than the situation warrants. In any case this is likely to be an inevitable stage since models will usually precede the completion of research designed to test them. (p.9).

Holden (1990) argues that while it may not be possible to test scientifically the underlying assumptions and propositions of nursing models it is possible to scrutinize certain aspects of nursing care affected by their introduction.

*Research into the effects of nursing models in mental health*

Acknowledging the lack of research on the effects of nursing models Chinn and Jacobs (1987) in the U.S. and Walsh (1989) in the U.K. recommend that investigations be carried out to determine the results of applying nursing models.

Webb (1986) states that until well planned evaluative research is carried out:

It will be impossible to say whether it is the individual skill, knowledge and sensitivity of a certain nurse or the use of a particular model which leads to the quality of care planned and given...until then we must rely on our own and others' subjective and impressionistic assessments of the benefits of using nursing models. (p.174).

Similarly Smith (1987) predicts:

It is possible that in ten years hence nurse educators will turn everything on its head and state that nursing models are a load of rubbish. However to do so may prove extremely difficult if no written record has been maintained with the explicit purpose of evaluating progress. (p.109).

Most of the available research into the evaluation of nursing models has used the survey approach and has been undertaken in North America. For instance Gordon (1984) employed anthropological methods of observations and interviews on two general surgical units to see if formal nursing models affected the way staff progressed from novice to expert. She found that models could be useful for new staff and students but experienced staff may find them too constraining and reductionist.

In one British study Keyzer (1985), a nurse tutor, used an action research approach to 'adopt' a nursing model in practice and education. He used the observer as participant role in four hospitals: one long-stay geriatric, one psychiatric rehabilitation, one community hospital and one psycho-geriatric assessment unit. His findings suggested that, in the absence of a redistribution of power and control from managers, educators and doctors to practitioners and patients, the change to a nursing model would be difficult. Keyzer also stresses the importance of education programmes to support the change. In essence therefore in order for the implementation of a nursing model to be successful the relationships between nurse, patient, relatives and managers would have to change (Keyzer, 1985).

In Canada the effects of the McGill University model of nursing have been appraised in clinical practice. According to Gottlieb and Rowat (1987) its use achieved the following patient outcomes: increased rates of satisfaction, decreased stress levels, increased problem solving and increased involvement in health learning. Ongoing evaluative research is also now being undertaken with the models of Roy and Orem (Fawcett, 1989).

Hoch (1987), using a quasi-experimental design, examined 48 retired individuals in Pittsburgh to see what effects the application of Roy's and Neuman's models would have on their rates of depression and life satisfaction. Findings were highly significant indicating that nursing care based on the two models resulted in lower depression scores and higher life satisfaction scores than did care based on no model of nursing. Hoch does accept that the personal characteristics of the nurses may have influenced the results and calls for the study to be replicated.

In a descriptive study Lerheim (1991) surveyed twenty eight experienced 'nurse leaders' in four Norwegian hospitals. Her goal was to see if nursing service used 'nursing science' to develop and improve practice. She found that the impact of nursing models was clearly expressed in a new independent attitude by practising nurses. Lerheim concluded that nursing models are being used directly and indirectly to make a difference to practice.

There is a dearth of research studies concerning the effects of nursing models on the care of individuals with mental health problems. Some psychiatric nurse researchers question whether models that have their roots in general nursing would have any positive effect on mental health care (Mason and Chanley, 1990). This view has also been expressed by Barker (1990) who, reflecting on the effects of applying nursing models to psychiatric care, stated that

> ...their value has not been demonstrated in research terms and some nurses have expressed reservations about the actual contribution to care made by nurses' use of such general nursing models. (p.342).

Most of the literature on the application of nursing models is composed of anecdotal care studies as opposed to rigorous empirical research. Nonetheless, there may be some benefits in examining practitioners' anecdotes about their experiences in applying models. Roper et al (1990) point out that feedback from practitioners using their model did provide the authors with a source of new ideas and highlight some of the application difficulties. Other theorists also found the anecdotal feedback from practising nurses helpful (Roy, 1980; Orem, 1980).

Involving practitioners in this way has other advantages. Firlit (1990) believes that taking the experiences of practising nurses into account is a vital link in establishing a 'theory-practice arena'. Chalmers (1989) argues that it is only by involving clinicians in assessing the worth of models that a firmer body of practice-related knowledge will be established. Therefore practising nurses must be involved in discussions about the application of nursing models. This is a valid strategy considering that it is the practising nurse who ultimately has to translate what Kuhn (1970) called the 'know that' of models into the 'know how' of practice.

# The effects of nursing models on quality of care

Most of the writers on quality assurance in health care cite Donabedian, an American physician, as one of their major influences. In 1966 he proposed that to examine the quality of service given by health professionals three distinct components should be focused upon. These were Structure, Process and Outcome.

*Structure* Structure refers to the resources and organization that are required as a basis for quality of care delivery. It includes numbers of personnel, their knowledge, their skill mix, equipment, buildings, finances, written policies and procedures.

*Process* Process is the doing part of a quality initiative. It is the action that the practitioner undertakes when giving care. Therefore it includes actions such as assessing, planning, implementing, evaluating, teaching, liaising and reassuring.

*Outcome* Outcome is the end product of the care delivered. It is normally patient and family centred and includes concepts such as patient satisfaction, patient knowledge, patient compliance and patient recovery.

Although Donabedian (1966) states that it is important to examine all three elements when looking at the quality of health care, there is no evidence to show that structure, process and outcome are significantly related. It is possible for patient outcomes to be poor despite good processes and good structural resources. Alternatively, some patients may get better despite poor processes of care. For instance Goffman (1961) found that many psychiatric patients improved in spite of hospitalization rather than because of it.

Zimmer (1974) advocates the appraisal of outcomes only. This is based upon the assumption that the desired end product of care is what is important. However this could be construed as ignoring the process of care delivery and lead to the accusation that the 'ends justifies the means'. Suchman (1967), in his acclaimed work on evaluative research, maintains that evaluation should include an examination of process and outcome. This has been supported by nurses like Bloch (1975) and Vaughan (1990). However, by taking this stance these authors could be accused of ignoring the importance of resources for quality of care delivery. If the structure is not examined, it cannot be determined if the resources had a favourable or unfavourable effect on the process of care or on the outcomes of care.

According to the World Health Organization (1985) the most important nursing goal of the 1990s is the assurance of quality of care. However in 1986 Pearson wrote that "A move towards model based practice is the most important target for change today.

It precedes all other innovations." (p.53).

What is the relationship between these two innovations? Does the application of a nursing model improve quality of care or does it cause such conceptual upheaval and confusion among practitioners that the quality of care suffers? It was possible to divide the literature regarding the perceived relationship into three main points of view:

1. nursing models lead to better quality of care;
2. an uncertainty as to the effect nursing models have on quality of care;
3. nursing models do not improve quality of care.

*Nursing models lead to better quality of care* Several writers offer the unsubstantiated opinion that using nursing models help improve the quality of care. For instance Fawcett (1989) writes that:

> It seems reasonable to expect that the use of models will foster a higher quality of nursing practice than is evident when an explicit model is not used to guide activities. (p.52).

Many respondents in part one of this present study maintained that the most positive aspect of nursing models was their ability to improve the quality of care (see table 5.12 p.69). McFarlane (1977), Green (1985), Herbert (1988), Hawkett (1989) and Melia (1990) have put forward similar opinions.

The most common argument to support these opinions appears to be that nursing models provide practitioners with a knowledge base on which to give care. According to Chalmers (1989) the development of nursing models is founded on a desire to provide high quality of care based upon an identified body of nursing knowledge. She continues by stating that a defined knowledge base for nursing should help to clarify the role of the nurse and provide a means of achieving high standards of care.

Other more specific reasons have been opined. Meleis (1985) argues that a model should improve quality because it clearly defines boundaries and goals, provides a guide to assessment, articulates nursing actions, provides continuity and congruency in care and allows for more accurate prediction of the range of patient responses and outcomes. Kershaw (1990) agrees, acknowledging that when practitioners use a nursing model there is little danger of them omitting vital aspects of intervention.

Similarly, Green (1985) believes that by using a nursing model practising nurses can find meaning in their work and so enhance their commitment and motivation - thereby

124

improving the quality of care. She also maintains that models may influence what nurses are taught, which is likely to influence what they believe they should be doing in their work and eventually what they do.

Other stated reasons for nursing models improving the quality of care include the opinions that they can be used to predict desired outcomes (Engstrom, 1984); that they will narrow the theory-practice gap (Kershaw, 1986); that they will lead to the actual setting of standards (Farmer, 1986); that they reflect individual differences in care (Chalmers, 1989); that they provide 'beginning criteria' for the evaluation of intervention outcomes (Fawcett, 1989); and that they will lead to improved use of nursing skills (Jones, 1990).

*Uncertainty as to the effect nursing models have on quality of care* Some nursing authors acknowledge that models have an impact on quality of care but they do not state whether the impact is positive or negative. For instance in 1986 Webb asked - can models have an influence on the quality of care? In 1988 Wright repeated Webb's question and in 1989 Fawcett and Carino commented noncommittally that "The use of conceptual models to guide nursing practice has a substantial and significant impact on the quality of patient care." (Fawcett and Carino, 1989 p.2).

In 1990 there were still nursing writers who would rather reserve judgment on whether the effects of models on quality was favourable or unfavourable. Walsh (1990) agrees that nursing models should improve care but he is not sure if they do. Cash (1990) merely presumes that the attempts to implement nursing models have "complex results" on the quality of care delivered.

*Nursing models do not improve quality of care* It is interesting that this viewpoint was not encountered very often in the literature. Although Green (1985) is credited above with seeing a positive link between models and quality she also acknowledged that it is possible that they do not improve the quality of care. She makes the proviso that it depends on the model used. An example of Henderson's model (1966) being applied in mental handicap is offered. Since this model has a physiological basis and mental handicapped people are not ill she believes it would improve the quality of care in a limited way only.

Gould (1989) warns that when a model is applied in a rigid manner standards of care could suffer. Further, she doubts that nurses can give high quality of care when they are stuck with a model that gives them no scope for innovation in caring. Collister (1988) also highlights the effects on care of applying models like "theoretical straitjackets". He points out that a nursing model in not a substitute for good nursing care and poor practice will not improve merely by using a nursing model.

125

*The relationship between models and quality: research evidence* Those authors who offer the second viewpoint above may be correct in being noncommittal. This is because to date there is very little empirical evidence to confirm or deny that nursing models have an effect on the quality of patient care. But if such research were available would its results be implemented by practitioners? Webb (1986) believes that:

> It would be naive and contrary to experience to think that if we had research evidence to demonstrate that using nursing models helped improve standards for patients and nurses alike, their implementation would be readily accepted by nurses in general. Nurses are no different from anyone else and evidence is not seen as sufficient reason for changing behaviour. (p.209).

Nevertheless Storch (1986) wrote that skeptics might find nursing theory somewhat more palatable if they can be convinced that its application to nursing can make a significant difference to the quality of patient care.

Gould (1989) suggested that a programme of quality assurance should be produced using a nursing model to generate standards of care. In a small study at Guy's Hospital, London, Brewster et al (1991) did just that. They used the 'activities of living' elements from Roper et al's (1980) model to write twenty nursing standards for a pediatric intensive care ward. Although strengthening the relationship this initiative does not establish a causal relationship between quality and models.

*Methods of organising nursing care*

The implementation of a nursing model in a long-stay psychiatric ward could be affected by how the staff organize their workload. A common advantage cited for using a nursing model is that it encourages individualized care and discourages the traditional task centred approach.

Towell (1975) identified different methods of delivering care in a psychiatric hospital. He found that on therapeutic community wards nurses did focus on patients' individual problems, on acute admission wards the medical diagnosis had an important influence on patient care and on psychogeriatric wards task oriented care was the modus operandi. Reviewing the general and psychiatric literature Miller (1989) noted that "practising nurses in long-stay wards see their work in terms of tasks, workload and work routines...." (p.48).

Research by Bowers (1989) and Armitage (1991) indicated that primary nursing led to better quality of care. Nonetheless, according to Drummond (1990), the most

126

common approach to organising psychiatric nurses' work is team nursing. However, he argues that it can encourage practitioners to adopt a bureaucratic cognitive style that constrains learning. He advocates that students of psychiatric nursing should be exposed to supervised primary nursing. In the present study it would be difficult to introduce a nursing model in an area where task orientation was the dominant method of work organization. The lack of individualized care inherent in such an approach would be at variance with the basic philosophy of the Human Needs model.

## Conclusion

It appears that the literature is replete with unsubstantiated opinions about the links between models and practice and between models and quality. Because the available research is small and inconclusive there are unrelenting calls for more studies into examining possible links between these components. However, throughout the literature authors and researchers were in agreement that models can and should be used in practice, and improvements in care are legitimate criteria for evaluating the worth of these models.

# 10 Literature review: change to model based practice

**The change process in applying nursing models**

> Change is not made without inconvenience, even from worst to better.
>
> (Johnson, 1734 p.91).

Kuhn (1970) theorised that as professions evolve they 'shift' from paradigm to paradigm as the needs and perceptions of society and the professionals themselves alter. A paradigm shift is a new way of looking at old situations. Psychiatric nursing is now passing through a paradigm shift. Professionals are changing their focus from a medical model towards a nursing model. It was pointed out in part one of this study that this paradigm shift is far from complete.

There may be some legitimacy in viewing Kuhn's theory in a slightly different way. Nurses who have been using a particular nursing model for a period may realize that it is not meeting the patients' care requirements. Others may have been using a nursing model improperly and as a result they are failing to influence patient care. Such insights may lead nurses themselves to seek a paradigm shift to another model thereby enabling them to work with patients from a more appropriate perspective. If over time the new model also fails to meet the requirements of practice a further paradigm shift may occur.

Johnson (1990) points out that paradigm shifts are often viewed as innovations simply because they challenge the present order. In their study Salanders and Dietz-Omar (1991) found that the introduction of a nursing model represented a change in the philosophical orientation of the nurse. Earlier Wright (1988) argued that change will occur in any setting where a nursing model is being adopted (p.155). On the authority of Robinson (1990):

The adoption of formal models is essentially a precursor to radical change. It is an explicit call to change practice.... That is why, of course, so many of the proponents of the use of models among practitioners are those who are at the forefront of change. They are those who care about the nursing practice which they can offer and are seeking ways to improve it. (p.11).

Therefore it is not surprising that the literature dealing with the introduction of nursing models into clinical practice tends to follow the various theories and strategies of change outlined above. However the first sentence in Robinson's quote can only be accepted with certain reservations. Without proper understanding and planning the adoption of model based practice will not be a precursor to radical change. Change to model based practice has often been introduced superficially while old practices endure (see Sternberg, 1986).

*Assessing the need for a change to a nursing model*

Applying a nursing model to practice is an undertaking that should only be approached after much preparation. Prior to its introduction it is important to make sure that the model is not going to replace a more appropriate one already in use. Therefore it is essential to find out how good or bad the previous formal or informal model of care is.

Most of the literature stresses that the introduction of a nursing model requires considerable time, dedication, commitment and support both moral and financial (Aggleton and Chalmers, 1990; Jones, 1990; Walsh, 1990). Therefore efforts should be made to ensure that all those who are going to be affected by the model including nurses, patients and their families understand its philosophy and find it acceptable. Further, the type of patients and their medical and nursing needs must be considered.

The responsibility, authority and autonomy of the practitioners are other important considerations. Vaughan (1990) believes that to introduce a model nurses have to have the freedom to manage their work and not be bound by the rules and regulations of a rigid hierarchy. Keyzer (1985) whose study has been referred to in chapter ten argues for a redistribution of power to patients and ward staff.

It may also be prudent to assess the attitudes that clinical staff and patients have towards nursing models and towards change. Sharp (1991) states that attitudes are precursors of behaviour and a person's attitude may constitute a predisposition to respond to something in a negative or positive way. So a negative attitude towards nursing models and an unwillingness to change may influence practitioners' motivation and the acceptance of the change.

Careful assessment of the environment is also important as ward layout can sometimes thwart attempts to implement a nursing model successfully (Jacox, 1974; Aggelton and Chalmers, 1990). However the resources required to make the environment more receptive to model based practice may be difficult to obtain when there are increasing financial restraints and when existing services are stretched to the limit.

Capers (1986) summarized the major assessments that must be made prior to introducing a nursing model:

> It is important to determine if the nursing practice environment is conducive to using the nursing model, what outcomes are anticipated for its use, which nursing personnel will use the model, how are staff to be prepared to use the model, how and when will the model be evaluated and the financial resources that are needed and those that are available.
>
> (cited in Fawcett, 1989 p.54).

*Planning the change to a nursing model*

According to Wright (1988) the power-coercive approach is not an appropriate change strategy for the implementation of a nursing model. If this is attempted he warns that a 'shifting sands effect' will occur with a reversion to old norms once the change agent moves on. He advocates Ottoway's (1976) 'bottom up' approach with an on-site change agent taking account of the views of clinical nurses.

Several authors suggest that the best way of introducing a nursing model is to use a few patients as a pilot group. This decreases the amount of 'future shock'. Future shock is "The shattering stress and disorientation that we induce in individuals by subjecting them to too much stress in too short a time." (Toffler, 1970 p.4). Using a pilot group also focuses the contributions of the practitioners involved (Dyer, 1990).

When planning change it is important to have a collaborative approach with all those affected being involved in the discussions. In their study into the use of Orem's model, Denyes et al (1989) found that communication was critical to the success of the venture. Frequent meetings of interested parties enhanced mutual understanding of the goals, plan, methods, problems and solutions. Discussions among participants were especially valuable for standardising the implementation approach. Chapman (1990) also stresses the importance of communications believing that:

> The ethical way to introduce a nursing model is to hold discussions with clinical nurses, managers and nurse educators so that they can decide for themselves

whether a particular nursing model merited experimental implementation. (p.14).

*Implementing the change to model based practice*

Some writers place the responsibility of implementing a nursing model solely in the hands of practitioners (McFarlane, 1986; Luker, 1987). However others suggest (as with the assessment and planning phases) a coordinated approach involving management, teachers and clinical staff working together over a substantial period (Johns, 1990; Walsh, 1990). The latter approach recommends that change agents create group situations that enable the staff to come together for mutual support and for democratic discussions on implementation problems.

Salanders and Dietz-Omar (1991) maintain that the first major step in implementing a nursing model is to have formal and informal educational sessions. This will help the ward staff to become familiar with the model and give them the skills necessary to apply it. According to Dyer (1990) this will make it meaningful to them and help to minimize their fears and anxieties about the new model.

As referred to in the previous chapter the model may have to be adapted to suit particular patient care problems and care planning documentation will have to be changed. When using the nursing process to apply a model Kershaw and Salvage (1986) stress that the difficulty of nurses identifying patients' needs that cannot be met must be addressed. They suggest that it is more realistic for the assessment to be directed "...solely and specifically to those patient needs that the nurse is able to meet through a constructive and achievable careplan." (p.xiii).

Critics of nursing models argue that in most areas where nursing models are introduced the documented care plan may have changed but the actual delivery of care has not (Sternberg, 1986; Luker, 1988). In the words of Vaughan (1990) "the change is only skin deep". Therefore although suitable documentation is important the model's philosophy must be reflected in the care carried out with patients.

*Evaluating the change to model based practice*

The dearth of research literature on the evaluation of models in practice has already been mentioned in the previous chapter. Researchers like Denyes at al (1989) give some guidance on what should be evaluated. They support Suchman's (1975) process-outcome approach to evaluation. However Walsh (1990) acknowledges that prior to doing this, reliable and valid tools must be formulated. He states that just measuring patient satisfaction is no longer appropriate.

131

## Lippitt's theory of change

Lippitt (1973) identified a seven step theory of planned change.

### Step 1 diagnosing the problem

This step provides the foundation for planned change. All participants involved in the proposed change should examine the situation and note whether the change is necessary. A perception of problems with the current situation is created and a change is seen as a worthwhile goal. In other words there is a 'felt need' for change.

### Step 2 assessment of motivation and capacity for change

In this step the commitment to change is assessed. Change is not an easy process and if there are many personal, organizational and environmental barriers to change the idea of implementing change at all may have to be reconsidered.

### Step 3 assessment of change agent's motivation/resources

It would be ethically improper for outsiders to identify a need for change and encourage others in that direction if they themselves were not enthusiastic for the change. If an internal change agent is to be involved he or she also must have as high a level of understanding, knowledge and motivation as the external change agent.

### Step 4 selecting progressive change objectives

In this step the planned change is implemented. Explicit objectives should be made regarding what has to be done, who should do what, how they should do it and when it should be done.

### Step 5 choosing the appropriate change agent's role

As referred to above (p.228) Ottoway (1980) sees the change agent as having many roles depending on the change that is to take place. Within Lippitt's theory they also may have a teaching input, be a group leader, an action facilitator, a catalyst or an expert role model. Regardless of the role taken all the participants involved in the change must have a similar perception of and agreement on the role.

### Step 6 maintenance of the change

After the change has been introduced it is important that the organization does not revert to old practices. Time is required for the change to become successfully integrated and fully accepted. The initial enthusiasm for the change seen in steps 2-5 may wane and the change agent(s) may have to remotivate participants.

*Step 7 termination of the helping relationship*

At some stage the external change agent has to withdraw and allow the participants to maintain ownership of the change. If organizational members have not been completely involved in the change process this termination could prove detrimental to the change. Also premature separation of the change agent may lessen the stability of the change. Leddy and Pepper (1989) point out that before termination an evaluation of the process and outcomes of change must take place. When successful termination is finally achieved the external change agent may act as an outside consultant and resource person for the organization.

## Change in long-stay psychiatric wards

> The nurse tells him no,... She tells him how the schedule has been set up for a delicately balanced reason that would be thrown into turmoil by the change of routines. (Kesey, 1962 p.97).

In the first part of this study the literature concerning long-stay mental health care is dealt with in some detail. It is proposed in this section to concentrate on how the introduction of change affects this type of patient.

In their study Lemmer and Smits (1989) state that "Notions of persistence and lack of change are basic to the definition of the long-stay, chronic or institutionalized person." (p.4). They believe that the reason for this lack of change is due to the alienation, despair, powerlessness and hopelessness that long-stay psychiatric environments encourage. Mental health care has been seen by some as the 'Cinderella' of the health service. Perhaps, because of their lack of resources, lack of trained staff and labels such as 'back wards' the long-stay wards in psychiatric hospitals may be seen as the 'Cinderella' of the psychiatric service. This image does not encourage positive change.

In discussing the introduction of change on long-stay psychiatric wards, Armitage and Morrison (1991) comment that such an endeavour is fraught with difficulties. They admit that these wards are full of chronic cases and since only the most basic aspects of care can be delivered poor staff morale and low motivation are common. This view has been supported by various research reports (Rhodes, 1985; Armitage, 1990). However findings from the study by Cope and Cox into four psychiatric wards

(1980) showed that the greatest changes occurred on the long-stay ward (see below). Improvements were noted in care planning, patients' hygiene, meal presentation and patients' independence. Therefore successful change can be achieved but there is broad agreement among researchers that it must be handled skillfully and sensitively (Towell and Harris, 1979; Nolan, 1989; Armitage and Morrison, 1991).

*Research into change in long-stay psychiatry*

An American study by Schuler and Campbell (1974) examined the process of change in a thirty nine bed open psychiatric ward. In an attempt to introduce a therapeutic community approach to care they applied the principles of planned change. This included the identification of the researchers themselves as change agents, participation of practitioners and regular democratic staff meetings. The researchers did experience some resistance from the psychiatrist but this was resolved after the benefits of the change were outlined.

Schuler and Campbell had weekly meetings with the patients to discuss their feelings about the change. They found that the patients initially expressed a reluctance to change. This was manifested in a lack of trust, fear of failure, extreme dependence on staff and stereotyped perceptions of care. However after patient-staff meetings were organized to give knowledge, support and direction the patients actively participated in the change.

In Britain Martin (1974) also successfully changed a traditional hospital (Claybury) into a therapeutic community using a longitudinal experimental design. Over a six year period he noted that there was a reduction in institutionalization and an increase in rehabilitation and resocialization. He found that the use of patient and staff meetings was fundamental to the change as such meetings were a forum for resolving tensions and anxieties concerning the change. Martin warns that meetings of this sort are unsuccessful if not supported by all the staff.

In the same year in the United States Fairweather et al (1974) undertook an extensive project where they tried to encourage a large number of psychiatric hospitals to create 'community lodges'. These may best be described as community residences functioning without staff and having a type of therapeutic community ethos. During the initial investigations the researchers gained valuable information on institutional practices and of the values and beliefs of the hospital staff.

Of the 255 hospitals approached only 23 attempted to develop 'community lodges'. Although this was disappointing to the researchers they did meet with a degree of success in the adoption of the innovation. In retrospect it is obvious that the project was too large and that Fairweather et al (1974) had difficulty controlling the many variables involved. Nevertheless for researchers interested in introducing change it has three valuable lessons; change agents are a precious resource, use a small number of pilot change areas and change requires considerable personal and persistent attention from the change agent.

In 1979 Towell and Harries wrote a book about their experience with implementing change in the Fulbourne Psychiatric Hospital in Cambridge. They used an action research approach to guide what was called the Hospital Innovation Project (HIP). The HIP began after a 1971 Hospital Advisory Service report recommended that behavioural science resources should be made available to staff in the hospital to facilitate change.

In the first two years of the project over twenty major and minor projects were initiated. The essential philosophy was that the hospital staff themselves played a leading role in these projects relying on the advisor for guidance. Some of the projects had a multidisciplinary input but most involved nurses. The change approach used by the project team was an amalgamation of 'bottom up' and a 'top down' approach with a greater emphasis on the former. A change agent could advise, support and guide but the onus for the change had to be from within the hospital. An 'Innovation Forum' composed of a cross section of staff members was set up. The results of the projects were mixed but a variety of identifiable innovations in patient care emanated from them. A summary of each project can be found in Towell and Harries (1979, p.202-212).

Cope and Cox (1980) successfully changed many different aspects of the care on four British psychiatric wards. These included changing managerial practices, improving multidisciplinary team work and improving the staff development service. They noted that Health Advisory Service reports told staff 'what they should do' but did not give any guidance on 'how they can do it'. Using a form of action research they involved practitioners in the change process. Regular meetings were held at ward level involving those affected by the change. The researchers believed that this helped to build up trust and generated a feeling of ownership among the participants for the change.

Also in Britain Cadbury (1980) described how she used a social ecological approach to change the atmosphere on a psychiatric admission ward. The study was in three distinct parts. Part one involved the application of Moos's (1974) 'real' and 'ideal' ward atmosphere scale to staff and patients. Part two involved the use of a weekly 'therapy group' where possible changes to the ward atmosphere were discussed and part three involved the reassessment of ward atmosphere six months after the initial

135

application. Findings from part three indicated that patients perceived the ward as significantly more oriented towards resolving their personal problems.

In a small British study Ward and Bishop (1981) attempted to measure the change in quality of care resulting from the introduction of the nursing process on two wards designated for the care of elderly mentally ill people. Using a quasi-experimental design the researchers identified a control ward where no change was to take place and a 'change ward' where the nursing process was to be applied. A pretest/posttest schedule was designed. The quality of patient care scale (QualPaCS) was used as a process oriented quality assurance measurement tool (Wandelt and Ager, 1974). Regular staff meetings were organized to gain support for the proposed change and to update staff on the progress of the change. The researchers gained the backing of senior nurse managers and involved nurse teachers in giving educational support. One year after the pretest measurements QualPaCS was applied for the second time. The researchers found a "considerable improvement in the 'change ward' with regard to individual and group interactions." (p.52).

In the United States Bevvino et al (1984) used a planned change approach to create a rehabilitation milieu for chronic psychiatric patients. Part of this change involved a progressive absence of nursing cover for the unit and the introduction of a self-medication programme. The 'locus of control' for the change was placed in the hands of four masters educated clinical nurses. These change agents started by educating the staff and patients towards the change. They felt it was important to have management support but more important to involve the staff and patients in the change process. After some initial 'struggles and challenges' the change was implemented successfully.

The study entitled 'Facilitating Change in Mental Health' by Lemmer and Smits (1989) was part of a Management of Change Project in a large Victorian psychiatric hospital in London. They used an action research design on five psychogeriatric wards. The study centred around the measurement of the change that takes place as a result of various educational inputs. Agreeing with the basic premise that "change goes hand in hand with learning" they used in-service education as a stimulus to change (p.17). As with most change projects of this kind in psychiatry the researchers used a 'bottom up' approach. This included the involvement of all those affected by the change, good communications through regular group meetings and the encouragement of ground level ownership of the change. The researchers adopted the philosophy of Towell and Harries (1979) who believed that the change should be from within and among the participants.

Lemmer and Smits (1989) monitored the effect of their change using Donabedian's structure, process and outcome approach to quality assurance. They recognized that "At some stage any project concerned with the management of change would have to include an evaluation of all three components." (p.97). During the change process they experienced uncertainty among staff. Comments such as "tell us what we are to do", "I don't know" and "show us", were common. Time had to be spent helping staff through these uncertainties. They also experienced active 'interference ' by organizational members in an attempt to sabotage the change. Some of this came from a small group of nursing officers who consistently disrupted the quality and continuity of care on the research wards by moving staff. Nurse educators also interfered with the change by continually requesting proof that the change was taking place.

Despite this uncertainty and interference Lemmer and Smits (1989) found the experience rewarding and developed what they referred to as a 'multifired engine' model for change. They also enabled the ward staff to communicate better, to develop quality circles and to write a patients' Bill of Rights that has laid the foundation for the formulation of standards for psychiatric care.

For his doctoral thesis Armitage (1990) evaluated the change towards primary nursing on a long-stay psychiatric ward in Wales. The study was in two parts. In the first part he undertook an exploratory study of the care setting, finding that the underlying philosophy for patient care was a custodial one. The second part involved the application of a triangulation of methods before and after the introduction of primary nursing (the planned change).

To prepare and support ward staff for the introduction of primary nursing, Armitage identified an internal change agent whom he calls the 'nurse preceptor'. However to obtain a setting conducive to change, alterations had to take place in the structural environment of the ward. Results show that the change to primary nursing increased the accountability and autonomy of the nurses. Further, the residents became more independent and self sufficient and the numbers moving to care in the community increased.

## The conceptual framework for this part of the study

It is proposed to facilitate the introduction of the Human Needs model on a long-stay psychiatric ward using an amalgamation of Lippitt's theory (1973) and Donabedian's (1966) taxonomy of structure, process and outcome (See figures 10.1).

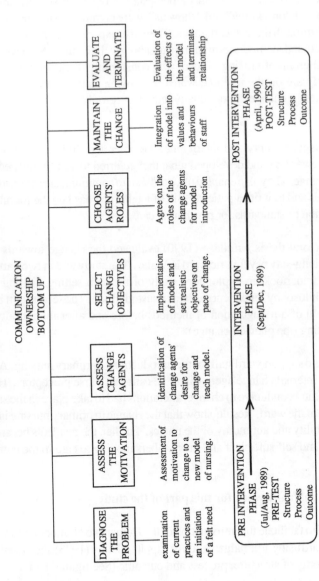

**Figure 10.1. The frameworks of Lippitt and Donabedian in relation to the phases of the present study**

COMMUNICATION
OWNERSHIP
'BOTTOM UP'

| DIAGNOSE THE PROBLEM | ASSESS THE MOTIVATION | ASSESS CHANGE AGENTS | SELECT CHANGE OBJECTIVES | CHOOSE AGENTS' ROLES | MAINTAIN THE CHANGE | EVALUATE AND TERMINATE |
|---|---|---|---|---|---|---|
| examination of current practices and an initiation of a felt need | Assessment of motivation to change to a new model of nursing. | Identification of change agents' desire for change and teach model. | Implementation of model and set realistic objectives on pace of change. | Agree on the roles of the change agents for model introduction | Integration of model into values and behaviours of staff | Evaluation of the effects of the model and terminate relationship |

PRE INTERVENTION
PHASE
(Jul/Aug, 1989)
PRE-TEST
Structure
Process
Outcome

INTERVENTION
PHASE
(Sep/Dec, 1989)

POST INTERVENTION
PHASE
(April, 1990)
POST-TEST
Structure
Process
Outcome

138

## Summary of the literature review for part two of the study

There is agreement in the literature that introducing a nursing model represents a major change for practitioners. However it seems that change may be anxiety provoking for most people and for nurses in particular. There is the danger that a new model of nursing may be perceived as a criticism of current practice. However its successful introduction is greatly enhanced if the assessment, planning and implementing of change involve those who are to be influenced by it. If this collaboration is not present there is the possibility that resistance to change may take place resulting in open rejection of the change and even sabotage of the innovation.

In summarising the research undertaken into change in mental health care it is possible to identify key guidelines for change. These include a bottom up approach with top down approval, the use of internal as well as external change agents, giving participants ownership of the change, giving educational input as a foundation for change, having regular group meetings, involving patients and diffusing the innovation from within the organization. These guidelines will be adhered to in the present study through the use of Lippitt's (1973) theory of change. This should ensure that the practitioners concerned possess the 'locus of control' and their 'learned helplessness' is reduced.

# 11 Methodology

In this part of the study it is proposed to evaluate the effects the use of the Human Needs' model (HNM) has on certain specified quality of care concepts. These are resources of care (Structure), nursing actions (Process) and the end results of care (Outcomes).

**Operational definitions**

Several relevant operational definitions have already been specified in chapter four. However there are other terms that require precise defining. The following definitions are entirely specific to this study.

*Quality of care*

The adherence to those structure, process and outcome criteria that have been identified as dependent variables within this study.

*Structure criteria*

The required personnel and environmental resources for the delivery of care as measured by the Armitage assessment instrument (AAI), ward atmosphere scale (WAS) and psychiatric ward monitor.

*Process criteria*

The action that the practising nurse undertakes when giving care as measured by analysing care plan goals and the psychiatric patient monitor (Meenz, 1989).

## Outcome criteria

Outcome is the end product of the care delivered as measured by various research instruments within this study: it includes patient satisfaction, nurse satisfaction, patient dependency levels, medication patterns, nurses attitudes to nursing models and nurse perception of patients' behaviour.

## Patient satisfaction

The attitudes and feelings that long-stay psychiatric patients have towards the nursing care they receive as measured by the patient satisfaction scale within psychiatric monitor.

## Nurse satisfaction

The attitudes and feelings that psychiatric nurses have towards the nursing care they deliver as measured by the nurse satisfaction scale within psychiatric monitor.

## Patient dependency

The categorization of patients into one of four levels of care as measured by the patient dependency scale within psychiatric monitor.

## Research hypotheses

For this part of the study certain hypotheses were formulated. The null hypothesis $(H_0)$ is normally stated so that its rejection would lead to the acceptance of an alternative research hypothesis. The following null hypothesis is concerned with changes in dependent variable scores *between* an experimental ward (Ward X) and a control ward (Ward Y) over the research period.

$H_0a$ Change scores in the dependent variables are identical between Ward X and Ward Y over the research period.

The alternative hypothesis to this is a directional one:

$H_1a$ Change scores in the dependent variables will be larger in a positive direction on Ward X compared to Ward Y.

Another null hypothesis was employed concerning changes in the dependent variables *within* Ward X and Ward Y over the research period.

$H_0b$ There will be no change in dependent variable scores on Ward X or Ward Y between pre-test and post-test.

The alternative hypothesis is also a directional one:

$H_1b$ Post-test scores for the dependent variables on Ward X will be larger in a positive direction than pre-test scores.

### Introduction to the research design

Fox (1982) believes that if data required to meet the aims of a study 'cannot be found in the past and do not exist in the present' then an experimental design must be used. Most experimental designs use an experimental and control group. These groups are as similar as possible except that the experimental group receives the input of an independent variable whose effect is to be studied. The groups are then assessed on specific predetermined factors called dependent variables.

Diers (1979) believed that experimental designs:

> ...offered the opportunity to invent a new way of working with patients (or resurrect an old way) and test it to see if it really achieves the predicted consequences in patient behaviour or welfare. (p. 165).

Cormack (1983) argued that it was time for psychiatric nurse investigators to leave descriptive research behind and use more experimental studies that could help show the relationship between nursing performance and positive patient outcomes.

True experiments must have three properties. These are the manipulation of the independent variable, the existence of a control group and randomization of subjects. However Polit and Hungler (1987) point out that in certain nursing situations it is either unethical or impractical to divide randomly subjects into an experimental group and a control group. In this situation they suggest that a quasi-experimental design (Q.E.D) may be used. They define a quasi-experiment as:

> A study in which subjects cannot be randomly assigned to treatment conditions, although the researcher does manipulate the independent variable and exercises certain controls to enhance the internal validity of results. (p.535).

Several important quasi-experimental studies do exist in nursing. In Britain Armitage (1990) used a quasi-experiment to evaluate the effects of changing to primary nursing on a long-stay psychiatric ward. Other quasi-experiments have been used to test the reputed advantages of patient allocation for organising nursing care (Auld, 1978; Chavasse, 1978; Bockholdt and Kanters, 1978; Metcalf, 1982). Most of these researchers used quality of care, nurse's job satisfaction and patient satisfaction as their dependent variables.

A review of several quasi-experiments in Cook and Campbell's (1979) book on the subject led to the selection of the 'nonequivalent control group quasi-experiment' as the most appropriate design for the present study. This design lacks randomization but involves the measurement of dependent variables on control and experimental groups prior to and following the introduction of an independent variable with the experimental group. Polit and Hungler (1987) believe that this type of quasi-experiment is a very strong one "because of its practicality, feasibility and, to a certain extent, the generalizability of the findings." (p 132).

A review of the literature showed a dearth of studies that used comparative or experimental designs to evaluate the effects of nursing models on patient care quality. The present study does attempt to do this; the independent variable being the use of the HNM, while the dependent variables are a range of quality of care indicators reflecting Donabedian's (1966) Structure, Process and Outcome approach to quality of health care.

However, because it was important to involve the patients and staff in the implementation of the selected model an action research approach was adopted for use within the quasi-experiment (See figure 11.1 below). According to Macleod-Clark and Hockey (1979) action research is the approach of choice when a researcher wishes "to evaluate the effects of a specific change involving the people who are part of the situation." (p. 20).

They believe that the main advantage of action research is that through participant involvement in the change the successful implementation of an innovation is encouraged. This approach relates well to Reason's (1988) 'co-operative enquiry' where "all those involved contribute to...the action which is the subject of the research." (p.1). Kent et al (1990) contend that it is only through participatory and collaborative research that the theory-practice gap will be bridged.

Webb (1991) showed that definitions of action research commonly emphasize the facilitation of change through involving and motivating participants in a given project. Because of this unique relationship she refers to action research as an "enabling science" (p.155).

The action research approach is closely related to theories of change. This is probably because it was Kurt Lewin (1946), the change theorist, who first described action research. Lewin's five steps of action research (analysis, fact finding, planning, execution and evaluation) are plainly reflected in Lippitt's (1973) framework of change (see p.138).

Most British psychiatric nurse researchers who have used the action research approach did so in order to introduce change in clinical settings (Towell and Harries, 1979; Lemmer and Smits, 1989). It has been suggested that action research is the approach of choice when the aim is to change to a more systematic way of delivering nursing care (Grypdonck et al, 1979).

However, one can ask if it is reasonable to use an action research approach within a quasi-experimental design. Hale (1991) states that the theoretical roots of quasi-experiments lie in positivism while according to Susman and Everad (1978) the action research approach (AR) has its roots in phenomenology. Table 11.1 is constructed from information derived from Susman and Everad (1978) and Macleod Clark and Hockey (1979). It shows an apparent incongruity between the designs concerning some central properties.

**Table 11.1. Design differences between quasi-experimental and action research approaches**

| Properties | QED | AR |
|---|---|---|
| Holds variables constant | yes | no |
| Introduces change | yes | yes |
| Actively involves subjects in change | no | yes |
| Can attempt to generalize from data | yes | no |
| Researcher is mainly detached | yes | no |
| Subjects are mainly units of study | yes | no |

It may appear that these two approaches are incompatible. However there have been several modifications of the true action research approach. For instance Chein et al (1948) identified diagnostic action research, empirical action research, participant action research and experimental action research. In participant action research there is only collaboration between researcher and subjects in diagnosing the need for change and planning the change. In experimental action research the researcher may only collaborate with the subjects in setting up an experiment to introduce change.

144

In the present study attempts were made to carry out an amalgamation of 'participant and experimental action research' where the researcher, as an external change agent, worked collaboratively with the subjects in identifying a need to change, how the change was to occur and in educating towards the change. However, as the study progressed, the internal change agents implemented the change and the researcher concentrated on taking an evaluative role.

Hockey (1982) believes that research into nursing often requires a mix of designs. This combinationist approach has also been called for by Corner (1991) and Morse (1991).

> Researchers who purport to subscribe to the philosophical underpinning of only one research approach have lost sight of the fact that research methodologies are merely tools, instruments to be used to facilitate understanding. Smart researchers are versatile and have a balanced and extensive repertoire of methods at their disposal.
>
> (Morse, 1991 p. 122)

Friedrichs (1979) argued that action research required an experimental scientific design to underpin it. This combination of action research with experimental research is not an uncommon methodological approach among nurse researchers in Britain (Tierney, 1973; Metcalf, 1982; Pearson, 1985; Armitage, 1990). These researchers wished to evaluate the effects of an innovation in practice and they realized that there would be a better chance of success if subjects were actively involved in the change. However it is interesting that none of these researchers discussed the possible philosophical incompatibility of these two approaches. Webb (1991) does attempt to address this issue. She sees action research as a method of carrying out 'critical science' whose goal is to focus on open, unconstrained communications between researcher and participant. As a research philosophy action research forms a bridge between the positivistic and interpretative approaches.

*Qualitative versus quantitative research*

Within the past few years there has been a trend among nurse researchers in Britain in valuing qualitative research and devaluing quantitative research (Kent et al, 1990). The former category is praised as a source of 'rich' data while the latter is criticized as too objective, unrealistic and merely an exercise in 'number crunching'. This has led to a polarization that is potentially detrimental to nursing research (Reimer, 1985).

Corner (1991) suggests that one way of merging qualitative and quantitative research is to use what Denzin (1970) refers to as triangulation. This strategy may best be understood if we use a nautical example. While out at sea ships' navigators may take their bearings from more than one point of land. This gives them a more accurate and reliable estimate of their position. In applying this principle to social research an investigator may use a triangulation of methods to study a particular phenomenon. An investigator can also use what Denzin refers to as investigator triangulation where individuals other than the researcher collect data. Both types of triangulation will be used in the present study. Morse (1991) warns that triangulation is not a technique to be used for reasons of convenience. It greatly increases the work involved in a study and increases the duration of a study.

Therefore, to meet the aims of part two of the study, a quasi-experimental design was used incorporating a control and experimental group with pre and post tests being carried out on specified dependent variables. Within this design the independent variable (the use of a nursing model) was implemented using an action research approach and triangulation was employed to collect the data.

*Selecting the data collection technique*

Questioning, structured observations and the analysis of written records were used to collect relevant data. Questioning as a data collecting technique has already been discussed in chapter five.

*Structured observation* In order to appraise whether the quality of the care environment changed over the research period observations of the ward 'structure' were necessary. The researcher and two external assessors had to complete observational checklists. These were the psychiatric ward monitor (Meenz, 1988) and the Armitage assessment instrument (Armitage, 1990) respectively. In addition some of the ward nurses were asked to observe their patients and complete the NOSIE (Honigfeld and Klett, 1965) and patient dependency instruments. Polit and Hungler (1987) refer to these types of observations as 'structured observations'. This means that the selection, observation, categorization, recording and encoding the phenomena of interest are already predetermined by the research instruments.

Polit and Hungler (1987) outline the advantages of using an observation technique. However they stress that objective observations may be threatened by the observer's attitudes, prejudices and emotions. Similarly what is observed may be affected by the observer's personal interest in the results or by their misunderstanding of what is to be observed. Polit and Hungler also relate how observational biases such as enhancement of contrast effect, central tendency bias, assimilatory bias, the halo effect, the error of leniency and the error of severity may distort what is reported as observed. The researcher discussed the possible threats to objective observation with

146

the external assessors and with those ward staff who were to complete the NOSIE Instrument.

*Record analysis* Extant records that are used for research purposes have been called 'secondary data' because they were not amassed with the research purpose in mind. This is in contrast to primary data from research interviews, questionnaires or observations. American academics Gleit and Graham (1989) admit that the use of secondary data is a valid means of enquiry but virtually untried in nursing research. However O'Neill (1984) states that nursing records have been used by researchers in two ways: as an indirect source of data on the nursing care given and as a direct source of data on nurse record keeping behaviour. The first usage forms an integral part of the data collection process for psychiatric monitor (for example, "Is there evidence in the nursing notes that the patient was assessed for orientation to time, place and person?").

Records were also referred to in the present study as a source of secondary data on nurse/patient ratios. It was also felt that aspects of patient improvement may be reflected in how their medication pattern changed over time. Most of the medications prescribed for the patients on both research wards could be subsumed into four categories: phenothiazines, anti-depressants, anti-parkinsonian and medications for physical problems. Therefore individual drug kardexes were monitored on both wards over the research period.

Meleis (1985) argues that nursing models help the nurse identify the goals of patient care practice (p.31). Therefore, it was decided to review the care plans throughout the research period to note the number, type and content of the written goals. A psychiatric nursing colleague post-coded goal types into categories and these were compared with the categories made by the researcher. These were: physical, psychological, social, medical, cognitive and safety. A possible flaw with secondary data is that the records may not be a true reflection of reality. Nurses may be very good at writing reports or care plans rather than being good at practice. The converse could also be true.

**The dependent variables and their measurement tools**

The research instruments used to measure the dependent variables are outlined in table 11.2. Their rationale for their inclusion, origin, content and reported reliability and validity are discussed below.

Table 11.2. The dependent variables for this study, their measures and the data collecting details

| | DEPENDENT VARIABLE | MEASURE OF DEPENDENT VARIABLE | DATA COLLECTED FROM | DATA COLLECTED BY | DATA COLLECTION TECHNIQUE |
|---|---|---|---|---|---|
| 1. | Quality of ward environment and atmosphere. | Psychiatric Ward Monitor. Moo's Ward Atmosphere Scale (WAS). | Environment/staff | Researcher. | Observation/Questioning |
| 2. | Quality of care resources. | Armitage Assessment Instrument. (AAI). | Patients and Staff. | Researcher. | Patient interview; Staff postal questionnaire |
| 3. | Quality of care delivery. | Psychiatric Patient Monitor. | Environment, staff and patients. | External assessors. | Observation/Questioning |
| 4. | Type, number and content of care plan goals. | Record Analysis. | Patients, staff and records. | Researcher. | Patient/staff interviews. and analysing notes. |
| 5. | Patient satisfaction. | Patient satisfaction Scale. | Care plans. | Researcher. | Analysing written plans. |
| 6. | Patient dependency. | Patient Dependency Scale. | Patients. | Researcher. | Interviewing. |
| 7. | Nurses' satisfaction. | Nurse Satisfaction Scale. | Patients. | Key nursing staff. | Observation/ discussion. |
| 8. | Patient evaluation by nurses. | Nurse Observation Scale for Inpatient Evaluation. | Ward staff. | Self report by staff | Postal questionnaire. |
| 9. | Nurses' attitudes to nursing models. | Attitudes to Nursing Models Questionnaire. | Patients. | Key nursing staff. | Observation/ discussion. |
| 10. | Patient medication Patterns. | Record Analysis. | Ward nursing staff. | Self report by staff | Postal Questionnaire. |
| | | | Medicine kardexes. | Researcher. | Analysing written notes. |

148

The hypotheses apply to most of these dependent variables. The exceptions are the quality of care resources (2) and the type and content of care plan goals (4). The nominal data obtained for these variables did not lend itself to hypothesis testing.

*Reliability and validity*

Most of the research instruments used have been tested for reliability and validity by their originators and by many researchers. These psychometric values will be alluded to as the various instruments are described. Even though it was beneficial to have these published values, it cannot be assumed that they are transferable. Therefore it was decided to calculate the reliability of these instruments as they applied to the respondents in the present study.

As reported in chapter five the reliability of a research instrument is concerned with the consistency or repeatability of the data collecting tool. Since the time factor militated against a 'test-retest' approach, Cronbach's alpha was used. This is a robust statistical test designed to estimate the reliability of a measure composed of several items (Polit and Hungler, 1987). Alpha is easily interpreted with ranges .00 to 1.0 indicating low to very high internal reliability respectively. Ferketich (1990) states that this is the preferred reliability measure because the respondent is not burdened with the completion of an alternate form, does not need to retake an instrument a second time, nor is the researcher required to deal with the arbitrariness of split-half procedures.

The validity of a research instrument relates to the ability of the data collecting tool to test what it is purporting to test. The validity of the research instruments used in this study has been well reported in the literature.

*The nurses' observation scale for in-patient evaluation (NOSIE)*

The nurse's observation scale for inpatient evaluation was developed in the USA by Honigfeld and Klett (1965) as a behaviour rating scale to measure therapeutic change in older hospitalized patients who have chronic schizophrenia. It draws on the skill of nursing staff who are usually in the best position to make unobtrusive observations of patient behaviour over a three day period. The NOSIE scale has six dimensions of which three are positive - social competence, social interest, personal neatness and three are negative - irritability, manifest psychosis and retardation.

The rationale for its use in the present study was based on findings from the literature. Philip (1973), a British psychologist, used the 30 item NOSIE to study the effect of introducing a rehabilitation programme into a long-stay psychiatric ward. He found that it was a valid and reliable instrument for assessing change over time in this type of setting. He also found it more reliable and valid than Wing's more widely used social withdrawal scale. Copeland and Wilson (1989), discussing the use of rating scales in British psychiatry, stated that the NOSIE scale has been used with all age groups and is of use in non-demented institutionalized patients.

The standard NOSIE scale has 80 items and the shortened version 30 items (the latter scale was used in the present study). Each item is related to an aspect of patient behaviour. Frequency of behaviour determines scoring with 0 = never, 1 = sometimes, 2 = often, 3 = usually and 4 = always. The resultant score determines the patient's placing on the six dimensions.

Honigfeld and Klett (1965) report that the reliability and validity of the scale was tested on 265 psychiatric patients whose mean age was sixty six and who had been in continuous hospitalization over twenty four years. They found that the average rater reliabilities for each dimension were: Competence .89, Interest .76, Neatness .83, Irritability .81, Manifest Psychosis .73, Retardation (depression) .74. Results of calculating Cronbach's alpha for the present study are similar: entire 30 item scale .66, Competence .78, Interest .86, Neatness .83, Irritability .71, Manifest Psychosis .41, Retardation .85. In his British study Philip (1977) also found the dimension Manifest Psychosis to be "...much less reliable than the others." (p.595). Therefore the findings pertaining to this dimension will be examined with this in mind.

*Ward atmosphere scale*

The WAS has been used since 1968 on both sides of the Atlantic to evaluate the atmosphere of inpatient psychiatric treatment environments. The original WAS was a 100 item true-false questionnaire that could be applied to patients and staff. However Moos (1974) was able to reduce the number of items to 40 without threatening the scale's reliability and validity. He states that the shorter form is especially useful in following changes in a programme over time. Although the WAS is American in origin, Moos tested it on psychiatric wards in Britain.

The rationale for using the WAS in the present study was based on the research literature's assertions that ward atmosphere is an important factor to consider when appraising the quality of psychiatric care (Cadbury, 1980; Armitage, 1990). According to Butterworth (1991) "the evidence of the impact of environment on the course of mental illness is strong." (p.240). Further it has already been pointed out in chapter four that much of the psychopathological behaviour exhibited by long-stay psychiatric patients was seen to be a result of their hospital surroundings rather than a manifestation of their illness.

A unique feature of this instrument is that it includes a real and ideal ward atmosphere profile. This is of use in the present study because the discrepancy between real and ideal scores observed in the pretest may be compared with the discrepancy score observed in the post-test. Hence any positive or negative variation in the gap between real and ideal over time can be noted.

The WAS may be completed by an interviewer or by the respondents themselves. It assesses the respondent's perception of treatment environment along three dimensions: relationship, personal development and administration dimensions. These three dimensions are made up of ten subscales: Involvement, Support, Spontaneity, Autonomy, Practical Orientation, Personal Problem Orientation, Anger and Aggression, Order and Organization, Programme Clarity and Staff Control.

In Britain Sudgen (1977) and Milne (1986) used the WAS in psychiatric settings and found it to be one of the most widely used and best validated scales available to monitor deliberate changes in therapeutic settings over periods of time. Moos (1974) established construct validity for the WAS through correlation with other established scales. He also calculated reliability coefficients ranging from .70 to .92 for patients and .78 to .96 for staff. The calculated Cronbach's alpha reliability coefficients for the present study are: Relationship dimension .82; Personal Development dimension .84; Administration dimension .68; alpha for entire scale .90.

*Psychiatric monitor*

Psychiatric monitor is an extension of the work carried out for the North West Nurse Staffing Levels Project (Goldstone et al, 1983). It has been produced in three versions, long-stay care, acute psychiatric and psychogeriatric and its publication was the culmination of a three year research project (Meenz, 1988). According to Meenz it was constructed against the 'backdrop' of Donabedian's structure, process and outcome criteria and involved the contribution of patients and nurses. At the time of the study it was the only British quality assurance tool available for the long-stay psychiatric patient population.

Extensive validity testing and testing for inter-rater reliability has occurred in psychiatric hospitals throughout England (Meenz, 1988). Items that had less than 80% agreement among a panel of psychiatric nurses were either rewritten or excluded. In 1990 Bentley and Boojawon used psychiatric monitor. They concluded that it was successful in measuring the quality of care offered to patients.

Psychiatric monitor is composed of five main parts. These are: patient monitor, ward monitor, patient dependency, patient satisfaction and nurse satisfaction

151

instruments. As these were all used in the present study they will be discussed separately.

*Patient monitor*

This is composed of 75 items divided into three subsections: care planning (29 items), physical needs of patients (13 items) and patients' psychosocial and spiritual needs (33 items). An index of quality may be obtained for each of these subsections and for the patient monitor as a whole. A 'yes' response scores one point, a 'yes sometimes' response scores half a point, a 'no' response scores zero points and a 'not applicable' response is not included in the calculations.

Within the present study internal reliability of patients' monitor using Cronbach's alpha gives the following results: care planning subsection .93; physical needs of patients subsection .64; and patients' psychosocial and spiritual needs subsection .87. The alpha score for the entire patient monitor was calculated at .94.

*Ward monitor*

This part of psychiatric monitor has 94 items and examines structural issues such as ward management and support services. It is composed of five subsections: evaluation of nursing care (13 items); ward procedures (21 items); administrative services (39 items); non-institutional methods (17 items); and nursing development (4 items). A ward monitor index score can be obtained by using the same scoring system as specified for Patients' monitor.

Results from applying Cronbach's alpha to the present data set indicate the following internal reliability coefficients: evaluation of nursing care .78, ward procedures .79, administrative services .68, non-institutional methods .67, and nursing development .65. The alpha score for the entire ward monitor was .91.

*Patient dependency form*

There has been much literature on the measurement of patient dependency (Ball and Goldstone, 1983; Luft, 1990). In her research Miller (1989) states that patient dependency is the outcome of interactions between the patient and the institutional environment. She believes that:

> Estimates of dependency which are based only on the patient's medical and physical condition are likely to be particularly inappropriate in units where patients are hospitalized for long periods. (p.87).

Within psychiatric monitor patient dependency is "the amount of nursing care time required by the patient" and represents more than just medical and physical components (Meenz, 1988; p 19). Four categories are identified, each one representing a step on a continuum from independence to dependence. Patients in category one are self caring and require minimal nursing intervention while category four patients need constant attention and maximum nursing intervention. Patients in categories two and three require regular and considerable nursing intervention respectively. Category two has been described as a "tendency to category one" and category three as a "tendency to category four".

Allocation to one of the four dependency categories depends on which of 35 'care factors' apply to the patient. According to Meenz these 'care factors' have been identified by many practising and experienced nurses. Each care factor is weighted and after the nurses select the 'care factors' they add up the weightings and obtain a patient dependency score.

*Patient satisfaction questionnaire*

Since the Griffith's Report (1984) highlighted the importance of consumerism in health care the concept of patient satisfaction has become an important part of quality assurance programmes. Over the years nurse researchers in the UK have devoted considerable attention to measuring patient satisfaction (Metcalf, 1982; Hurst, 1988). However there have also been many authors who argue that patients seldom like to complain or appear dissatisfied with nursing care. This may be the result of the 'halo effect' towards nurses or fear of retaliation by nurses against those who complain. A good insight into this and other limitations of patient satisfaction surveys can be found in Ventura et al (1982) and LaMonica et al (1986).

There have been several British research studies on patient satisfaction with psychiatric care (Raphael, 1978; Armitage, 1990). In a review of the UK studies Altschul (1983) found that:

Patients are appreciative of nurses who listen, who are interested in what may appear to be trivial concerns, who have time for them and are available to join in activities and are friendly and accepting. (p.180).

In psychiatric monitor the patient satisfaction questionnaire is composed of 23 questions in five sections. The sections are: patients' wellbeing (4 items), information received (6 items), physical care (5 items), treatments (3 items) and ward staffing (5 items). Each question can have four potential responses: very satisfied; fairly satisfied; not really satisfied; and not at all satisfied. Scoring involves giving 3 points to a 'very satisfied' response, 2 points to a 'fairly satisfied' response, 1 point to a 'not really satisfied' response and 0 points to a 'not at all satisfied' response. Questions that are not answered are removed from the scoring system. From responses in the present study a Cronbach's alpha of .83 was calculated.

*Nurse satisfaction questionnaire*

According to McClune (1986) theories of job satisfaction have shifted their emphasis from bureaucratic values, that assume that people dislike work and will avoid it if possible, to a more democratic orientation that assumes that people like and seek fulfilment from their work. McGregor (1960) described these two approaches as Theory X and Theory Y. In 1974 Campbell et al argued that theories of job satisfaction and the related concept of motivation can be categorized as process or content theories. Process theories include expectancy theory and equity theory while content theories include the work of Maslow (1954) and Herzberg (1968). Campbell et al (1974) gives an excellent overview of these theories.

Herzberg's Motivation-Hygiene theory fits well with the nurse satisfaction questionnaire within psychiatric monitor. From studying 203 engineers and accountants Herzberg (1968) maintained that job satisfaction comes from factors intrinsic in the work ('motivators'). These include not only the work itself but the achievement of targets and the actual performance of tasks. Extrinsic factors ('hygienes') include working conditions, staffing and work schedules. According to Herzberg the 'motivators' bring job satisfaction and improve performance while the 'hygienes' help prevent job dissatisfaction and poor performance.

In Britain Vousden (1986) reported from a 'MIND' conference that psychiatric nurses are dissatisfied with what they can do with patients in hospital especially within a mainly medical model. There are several subsequent British studies that have examined aspects of psychiatric nurse satisfaction (Jones, 1988; Humphris and Turner, 1989; Armitage, 1990; Parahoo, 1991). Landeweerd and Boumans (1988) conducted a nurse satisfaction study in three psychiatric departments in Holland. They found that nurses on the admission wards had the highest satisfaction scores, nurses on short-stay wards had the lowest satisfaction scores while nurses on long-stay wards had an intermediate score. In explaining the latter finding the researchers state that nurses on long-stay wards do not have the higher expectations found among nurses on short-stay wards.

In psychiatric monitor for long-stay wards the nurse satisfaction questionnaire is designed to assess the ward staffs' perception of the quality of care being provided to patients. It also seeks views on the effect that numbers, mix and deployment of

154

nursing staff have on patient care. The instrument has the same five sections as the patient satisfaction questionnaire with identical response categories and scoring system. This enables easy comparison of data between both tools. From responses in the present study a Cronbach's alpha reliability coefficient of .72 was obtained.

*The Armitage assessment instrument*

This is a research instrument formulated by Armitage (1990). He used it to gauge the quality of care on two British long-stay psychiatric wards before and after primary nursing was introduced. To design the 155 item instrument Armitage compiled and adapted "three well proven checklists" (Elliot, 1975; Nodder, 1980; Raphael, 1978). Armitage states that assessors using this instrument can collect the data by observing the environment of care and by obtaining information from patients, staff and records.

The instrument is divided into 22 sections. The length of these sections range from 'Physical conditions in which residents live' (20 items) to 'Religious beliefs' (2 items). To score the instrument Armitage suggests that one point is given for a yes response and zero for a no response. Most of the items reserve a space for assessor's comments. If the response is yes with a favourable comment this item is scored 1.5. If the response is yes with an unfavourable comment this item is scored 0.5. Although Armitage does point to the valid origins of his scale he does not expand on other psychometric details. In the present study a Cronbach's alpha reliability coefficient was calculated at .93.

*Attitudes to nursing models scale*

According to the literature an acceptance of nursing models requires not only a change in practice but also a change in attitudes (Walsh, 1990). A comprehensive review of attitudes towards nursing models was presented in part one of this study. Baron and Byrne (1984) define attitudes as "Relatively lasting clusters of feelings, beliefs and behaviour tendencies directed toward specific persons, ideas, objects or groups." (p.126). They felt that our attitudes determine how we interpret and react to various situations and they exert powerful effects upon our overt actions.

Since Baron and Byrne (1984) argue that attitudes affect behaviour it was important to try to gauge the baseline attitudes of nurses on the research wards to nursing models and to assess if and how their attitudes change over the research period. However a review of the extant literature did not uncover a suitable research instrument. Therefore, with the permission of the authors, the attitude scale for the nursing process by Bowman et al (1983) was adapted for use within this study.

The instrument is a twenty item Likert-type scale with ten positive and ten negative statements reflecting most of the attitudes to nursing models reported in the literature. Each statement may be allocated a score of 1 to 5, with 5 reflecting a very positive attitude and 1 reflecting a very negative attitude. By totalling the 20 items an attitude towards nursing models score can be obtained. Bowman et al (1983) claim a reliability coefficient of .93 for their scale. In the present study an alpha reliability coefficient of .78 has been calculated. Furthermore, since the content reflects the attitudes expressed in the literature, the minimum of face and content validity can be claimed (Fox, 1982).

## Ethical issue

Official ethical approval for the study was obtained from the University of Ulster Ethical Committee. In addition there was to be concentration on the following: no involvement without knowledge and informed consent, voluntary participation with no coercion, no exposure of the subjects to mental stress, no invasion of privacy, a demonstration of respect to subjects, confidentiality, an assurance of investigative competence and integrity of the researcher and respect for a refusal to participate.

There are specific ethical issues relating to those experimental designs where one group gets a different treatment than another group. For instance it has been suggested that benefits should not consciously be withheld from a control group. It could be argued that this occurred in the present study. However there was no hard empirical evidence to suggest that nursing models were beneficial or harmful. If results should show that the model does improve quality of care then it can be introduced in the future to benefit the control group. Therefore a 'risk/benefit' decision was taken based on the belief that the potential benefits of the research findings outweigh the delay in the model's introduction onto the control ward.

Clarke (1991) states that particular attention must be paid to ethical issues when carrying out research with psychiatric patients. In the present study most patients were able to give informed consent themselves. However in five instances consent was obtained from the patients' families. For two patients (who had no relatives) the ward manager and doctor gave the informed consent. Subjects were required to give verbal rather than written consent for several reasons: some of the patients could not write; the study did not involve risk to the subjects; and simply agreeing verbally may not be as threatening to some patients as signing an official form.

## The hospital setting: selection, access and description

By a process of simple random selection Hospital A was chosen. Following proper research protocol the research proposal and a letter requesting permission to proceed was sent to the relevant senior nurse management. They agreed to support and co-operate with the request. Permission was also obtained from the Director of Nurse Education and from the hospital medical staff.

Hospital A is situated in spacious, well maintained grounds three miles outside a major city in Northern Ireland. It is a modern building consisting of nine separate villas and an admission block. It was officially opened in 1961 replacing the old Victorian city asylum. Its catchment population is approximately 240,000. Like most large psychiatric institutions, over the past twenty years the hospital has been gradually reducing its in-patient population. In 1969 this numbered 735. At the start of the study (July 1989) there were 471 beds with inpatient numbers fluctuating around 370.

The National Unit for Psychiatric Research and Development (London) undertook a study of hospital A in 1989. They found that there were 188 patients whose length of stay was greater than 6 months and who did not have a primary diagnosis of dementia. Their mean length of stay was 18.4 years and 50% were over 60 years of age. Two thirds had been diagnosed as suffering from schizophrenia and over half of these had been assessed by medical staff as having 'low', 'very low' or 'poor' levels of social functioning. Around 30% of the long-stay patients were rated as particularly hard to place in the community with 26% being recommended for permanent hospital care (N.U.P.R.D., 1989).

*The research wards: selection, access and description*

Within Hospital A the long-stay area is composed of 11 wards architecturally structured into six distinct villas. In June 1989 one ward (Ward X) was picked at random from this sampling frame to be the experimental ward for the study. At a nursing staff meeting it was explained that the researcher wished with their permission and involvement to facilitate the introduction of the HNM to the care of patients on the ward. The findings from part one of the study were discussed. It was pointed out that a range of evaluative measures would be taken at various stages during the nine month period that the study would last. It was also explained that, although he had experience introducing nursing models into psychiatric practice, the researcher had never used the HNM.

The researcher then discussed the study at a patients' meeting. It was explained that their permission would be sought not only to answer questions but to consult their nursing notes. The ethical aspects of the study were described. They were also told that they could see the researcher's notes at any time and they could opt out of the study if they wished to do so. Both patients and staff were then given one week to decide if they wished the research to proceed. Before this period had elapsed contact was made to say that the patients and staff had given their consent to participate in the study.

The next stage in the project involved matching this ward with another long-stay ward in the hospital. This second ward would be the control ward and be called Ward Y. The matching criteria included: patient numbers, patient sex, staff numbers, staff mix, qualifications of staff, nurse management, organization of patient care and medical and paramedical input. This was achieved and a similar process of discussing the proposed project with Ward Y's staff and patients was undertaken. It was pointed out that although no change was to occur on Ward Y the researcher would be spending the same amount of time there as he was on Ward X. The staff and patients expressed an interest and gave their consent for the study to proceed.

The researcher had to work abroad for one month and on his return all the patients had been transferred from Ward Y to a variety of wards throughout the hospital. Other patients had been transferred into Ward Y and two of the matching criteria with Ward X (gender and consultant) could not now be met. Nevertheless after much discussion with nurse management it was decided that Ward Y was still the closest match for Ward X within the hospital. Permission was sought and gained from the new patients and staff on Ward Y. Figure 11.1 shows how both wards were incorporated within the research design.

Both wards formed a single structural unit, with Ward X constituting a mirror image of Ward Y. As a whole the unit will be called Apple Villa. Both wards were approved by the Northern Ireland National Board of Nursing, Midwifery and Health Visiting (NINB) as suitable for training student nurses for part three of the register. Both wards also shared the same clinical teacher and nurse tutor.

Although the research wards had access to a multidisciplinary team (including psychiatrists, physiotherapists, occupational therapists, social workers and psychologists), staff admitted that there were seldom any team meetings. Throughout the nine month period of the study there was no evidence of multidisciplinary meetings on either ward. Each research ward had one psychiatric consultant and a senior house officer. A medical ward round was normally held on a Wednesday or Thursday morning. There was a small social therapy unit staffed by two nurses near the villa. They had an input on both wards where they undertook patient discussions, groupwork and cookery classes.

**Figure 11.1.   diagrammatic representation of the research design**

POPULATION
All Long Stay Wards In Hospital A

Ward X 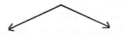 Ward Y

| PRE-TEST | PREINTERVENTION | PRE-TEST |
|----------|-----------------|----------|
| Specified |  | Specified |
| structure, |  | structure, |
| process and |  | process and |
| outcome |  | outcome |
| dependent |  | dependent |
| variables |  | variables |

INTERVENTION                                                      No Intervention
INDEPENDENT VARIABLE
(HNM) Using Action Research.

| POST-TEST | POSTINTERVENTION | POST-TEST |
|-----------|------------------|-----------|
| Specified |  | Specified |
| structure |  | structure, |
| process and |  | process and |
| outcome |  | outcome |
| dependent |  | dependent |
| variables |  | variables |

The organization of nursing care delivery on both wards was described by the ward managers as a combination of task allocation and patient allocation. A 'key nurse' system was in operation. This is a form of patient allocation where a member of staff is responsible for a small group of patients. Although there tends to be consistency in the allocation of nurse to patients the staff do not have 24 hour responsibility and accountability. This ultimately rested with the ward sister/ charge nurse.

According to the staff the nursing process was being used within Orem's self care model. However a National Board Inspection Report of the research hospital (NBNI,

1987) stated that:

> In many cases nursing assessments are almost exclusively dependent upon medical assessment and ...the identification of nursing problems are heavily medical model and physical condition orientated and even when nursing problems are identified they are generally unprecise or global in nature...In association with these difficulties there are also difficulties related to the use of a conceptual model in association with the nursing process. (p.12).

The report also states that "procedures are carried out routinely on the basis of traditional practice." (p 17). Preliminary investigations showed that this was still the case on the research wards when the present study was commenced.

## Patients' sample

Ward X had a complement of 20 beds and an average bed occupancy of 18 female patients. The mean age of patient was 71.38 years (S.D. 8.32 years; minimum age 59 years, maximum age 89 years). The mean length of stay (since last admission) was 17.94 years (S.D. 13.93 years; minimum stay 3 years, maximum stay 47 years). Although Ward Y also had a bed complement of 20, the average bed occupancy was 14 male patients. The mean age of patients was 64.2 years (S.D. 11.68; minimum age 40 years, maximum age 80 years). The mean length of stay was 17.5 years (S.D. 17.75; minimum stay 1 year, maximum stay 52 years).

**Table 11.3. T-test results showing how the research wards compare for patients' age and length of stay**

| Patient details | t-test result |
|---|---|
| Patients' age | $(t = 1.91, df = 29, p > 0.05)$ |
| Length of stay | $(t = 0.20, df = 29, p > 0.05)$ |

It can be concluded from table 11.3 that for age and length of hospital stay both wards were not statistically different at the 0.5% level of significance. The patients' daily routine was the same for both wards (See table 11.4)

### Table 11.4 Patients' daily routine in Apple Villa

| Activity | Time |
|---|---|
| Awakened | 8.00 - 8.30 a.m. |
| Breakfast | 8.30 - 9.00 a.m. |
| Lunch | 12.00 -12.30 p.m. |
| Snack | 3.00 - 3.15 p.m. |
| Tea | 5.30 - 6.00 p.m. |
| Supper | 7.00 - 8.00 p.m. |
| Latest bed time | 11.00 -11.30 p.m. |

Some of the patients attended social and industrial therapy departments in the morning and afternoon, returning to the ward for mid-day and evening meals. The evening period was seen as a period of relaxation where the patients watched television, played games, read or otherwise occupied themselves as a matter of personal choice. Personalized clothing and laundry facilities were available to both groups of patients.

Furthermore the patients on Ward X and Ward Y had similar psychiatric and physical diagnoses (See table 11.5).

### Table 11.5 The psychiatric and physical diagnoses of patients on both research wards

| Diagnosis | WARD X (n = 18) | WARD Y (n = 14) |
|---|---|---|
| Schizophrenia | 9 | 7 |
| Depression | 8 | 5 |
| Low I.Q. | 1 | 2 |
| Eye problems | 1 | 1 |
| Arthritis | 2 | 1 |
| Diabetes | 1 | 2 |

Since an essential part of the research involved asking patients questions, the issue of their communication abilities was an important one. Information from the staff and from patient records showed that there were two patients on each ward whom on occasions may not be willing or able to participate. This was due to them having periods of muteness or high excitability. Therefore when the term 'patients' is used in this thesis it refers to those residents on both wards who were willing and able to participate in the study.

**Staff sample**

All the nursing staff on both research wards were included in the staff sample. These comprised both day and night staff and included grades from ward sister/charge nurse to nursing students and auxiliaries. The 'day staff' worked 37.5 hours per week normally as 3x12 hour and 1x6 hour shifts per week. These shifts were an 'a.m.' shift (7.45 a.m.- 1.45 p.m.), a 'p.m.' shift (1.15 p.m. - 8.00 p.m.) and a 'long day' shift (7.45 a.m. - 8.00 p.m.). Night staff worked a 7.55 p.m. - 7.45 a.m. shift four nights one week and three nights the next.

Daily staff numbers and skill mix for Ward X and Ward Y are outlined in tables 11.6 and 11.7 respectively.

**Table 11.6 Daily staff numbers and skill mix on Ward X including daily averages over the nine month research period**

| Grade | Total | Day duty | Night duty |
|---|---|---|---|
| Ward sister/ Charge nurse | 2 | 2 | - |
| Staff nurse | 5 | 4 | 1 |
| Enrolled nurse | 1 | - | 1 |
| Student nurse | 4 | 4 | - |
| Nurse auxiliary | 1 | 1 | - |
| Totals | 13 | 11 | 2 |

| | Staffing quota | Daily mean no of staff over 9 mth research period |
|---|---|---|
| Qualified staff | 61% | 4.3 |
| Student nurses | 31% | 3.4 |
| Nursing auxiliaries | 8% | 0.4 |

**Table 11.7   Daily staff numbers and skill mix on Ward Y including daily averages over the nine month research period**

| Grade | Total | Day duty | Night duty |
|---|---|---|---|
| Ward sister/ Charge nurse | 2 | 2 | - |
| Staff nurse | 4 | 3 | 1 |
| Enrolled nurse | 1 | - | 1 |
| Student nurse | 4 | 4 | - |
| Nurse auxiliary | 2 | 2 | - |
| Totals | 13 | 11 | 2 |

| | Staffing quota | Daily mean no of staff over 9 mth research period |
|---|---|---|
| Qualified staff | 54% | 4.3 |
| Student nurses | 31% | 4.2 |
| Nursing auxiliaries | 15% | 0.6 |

The t-test for independent groups was used to investigate the relationship between the mean numbers of different types of nursing staff on both wards over the research period.

**Table 11.8   T-test results showing how the research wards compare for numbers of staff**

| Grade | t-test result |
|---|---|
| Trained staff | $(t = 1.00, df = 8, p > 0.05)$ |
| Student nurses | $(t = 1.58, df = 8, p > 0.05)$ |
| N. auxilaries | $(t = 1.00, df = 8, p > 0.05)$ |

Results show that during the research period there was no statistical difference between the numbers of staff on Ward X and Ward Y at the 5% alpha level.

The students on both wards were transitory subjects. They were mostly second and third year registered mental nursing (RMN) students whose ward allocation varied from nine to twelve weeks. The implications of this short allocation period will be discussed later. Ward Y had one male charge nurse and two male staff nurses. The rest of the staff on both wards were female.

## Pilot study

In her study Metcalf (1982) warns of the difficulties in undertaking a pilot study when an experimental longitudinal design is being used. This is because a pilot study would have to be as long as the main study itself. Despite this warning it is possible to use a pilot study to test the feasibility of the project, the research instruments, the data collecting methods and the data analysis plan.

In late July 1989 a pilot study was carried out on an adjacent long-stay ward (Ward W). This ward was a twenty bed long-stay female facility within the study hospital. Unlike the research wards it had some younger patients. Three older patients were selected by the ward manager and their permission was obtained; two staff members (one student and one staff nurse) were also included. A random sample of three nursing records and three medicine kardexes were also examined.

The pilot study lasted one week and the results indicated that the published research instruments were easy to apply, score and analyse. The project was feasible but some minor changes had to be made based upon the results. A change was made from the 80 item to the 30 item NOSIE. This was because the former was too long. Two nurses rating the NOSIE and the patient dependency levels independently of each other got remarkably similar scores. However this could be a long process and in the main study it was proposed to still use two raters but to have them working jointly.

The pilot study also showed that some of the items in psychiatric monitor were not specific enough. For example in the section dealing with admission there were questions regarding the initial assessment of the patient and who accompanied them to the hospital. These items were inappropriate considering that the mean length of patient stay was over 17 years and since nursing assessment notes then were almost non existent. Therefore it was decided to answer these questions from records now in use.

The pilot group also gave the impression that the respondents were trying to please the researcher. It was felt that this problem could be overcome in the research wards because a greater amount of time was to be spent there and hopefully the patients' desire to please the researcher would be lessened.

## Data collection procedure

The data collection procedure will be outlined in three distinct phases. These are preintervention, intervention and postintervention. The relationship of these three phases with the pre-test/post-test points and with Lippitt's seven step change theory is illustrated in figure 10.1.

*Pre-intervention phase*

In early August 1989 a period of two weeks was spent on both Ward X and Ward Y to observe the routines of care and to get acquainted with patients and staff. This was also an attempt to lessen the 'Hawthorne effect'. In mid August 1989 the process of collecting pretest baseline data on all the dependent variables was begun. The data that required minimum contact with patients and staff were collected first. It was hoped that this would give the patients and staff extra time to get used to the researcher's presence prior to their direct participation. Therefore data were initially collected from the ward environment using the psychiatric ward monitor and the Armitage Assessment Instrument.

The Armitage assessment instrument (AAI) was applied to the experimental and control ward by two external assessors. Both had many years experience working as psychiatric nurses and were at the time undertaking a research methods unit as part of their nurse tutors course. Neither assessor had worked in or had any connection with the study hospital. Due to pressure on their time they had not participated in the pilot study. However the researcher had piloted the AAI and so he spent three days with the assessors taking them through its application and scoring. Each item in the instrument was reviewed to ensure that both assessors had a similar understanding as to the meanings. They agreed to follow the ethics underpinning the study.

The external assessors were not told what the independent variable was nor which ward was the experimental ward or which was the control ward. They were asked not to seek this information and staff and patients were asked not to divulge it to them. After being introduced to the staff the assessors, equipped with an AAI for each ward, collected the data. They were asked to return the completed instruments to the researcher. The entire process lasted one day.

When these data were acquired all the nursing staff (n = 26) were given the ward atmosphere scale, the nurse satisfaction questionnaire and (excluding the three auxiliaries) the attitudes towards nursing models scale. A personalized letter was included reiterating the reasons for the study. Each staff member had a code number as a safeguard in case their completed questionnaire was misplaced and as a guide for analysis. The respondents were asked to return the completed instruments to the researcher via the hospital's internal mail system using the envelope provided.

It was recognized that nurses with responsibility for individual patients could be biased in their perception of their patients' abilities. To reduce this possibility key workers on both wards (n1 = 4, n2 = 4) were asked to work in pairs and complete the 30 item NOSIE and the patient dependency form for their patients. Most of completed instruments were returned within one week. The response rate for all staff instruments was 100%.

At their weekly meeting the patients were reminded that the researcher would be seeing them individually to ask them some questions. A letter confirming this intention was given to each patient. The WAS and the patients' satisfaction questionnaire were completed using a face to face interview technique. The researcher read out the questions and the patient answered with yes or no responses. Each patient was given a code number the key of which was known only to the researcher. The interviews lasted approximately fifteen minutes and were held in the wards' visitors' room. Two patients from Ward X and two patients from Ward Y decided not to take part. One of these ended their participation in mid interview.

A conscious decision was taken not to examine or analyse the pre-test or post-test data until after the researcher had completely finished the fieldwork. It was realized that this is a departure from the true action research approach where there is an ongoing sharing of the evaluation results with the subjects. However in this study it was judged unhelpful for the researcher or for staff and patients to know their scores. For instance, to be aware of the pre-test findings from either ward could result in increased effort or increased apathy by any of the above.

By the end of August 1989 the pre-test data were collected and the process of changing to the HNM was commenced on Ward X. Although the following report concerns Ward X the researcher spent a similar amount of time on Ward Y. Obviously it was important not to introduce any change on the control ward. Therefore the time was spent simply observing care and talking to staff and patients. It was not long before the researcher was fully accepted and could enter and leave almost unnoticed.

*Planned change*

*Step one* According to Lippitt's theory the first step in initiating a planned change is to examine collaboratively current practices and, if desired, initiate a 'felt need' for change (see chapter 10). It was obvious that the staff on both wards had been pressurized into using Orem's self care model. This model tended to reside in the ward office having a minimal influence on the care of patients. Literature on Orem's model featured prominently on the wards' notice boards. However the medical model tended to be the basis for many nursing practices with the medicine round and the doctor's round holding a prominent position in the wards' routines.

Because of the perceived shortcomings of Orem's model the initiation of a felt need for change on Ward X was easy to accomplish. A meeting was held with the nursing staff where they admitted that "trying to use Orem in practice felt like forcing a square peg into a round hole." Furthermore because of the results from part one of the study the staff felt the implementation of the HNM would be a worthwhile goal.

*Step two* Following Lippitt's second step for planned change an in-depth assessment of the motivation for change was undertaken. Each member of staff (including night staff, student nurses and nursing auxiliaries) was seen individually to determine their level of enthusiasm about the proposed change. A minority were unsure about their role within the research and expressed a lack of confidence in their capabilities. However they believed that the transition would be easier if a collaborative approach to change was adopted.

The motivation for the change among senior nurse managers was good. They agreed to give the ward staff autonomy and responsibility for the planned change and limit hierarchical interference. However they did say that if staffing numbers in other areas were to fall below safe levels nurses may have to be moved from the research wards for 'covering' purposes. But they did agree to treat Ward X and Ward Y equally in this respect. A second meeting with the two psychiatric consultants showed that they continued to endorse the change but had no desire for active involvement. From talking to the patients it was discovered that none were aware that Orem's model had been in use on the ward. Although they were unsure of what benefits the HNM would have for them they also gave the change their support.

There appeared to be no resistance to the change. Being familiar with the literature the researcher found this surprising. One possible reason may have been that the ward staff had implemented a model before (Orem's self care model) with no support or education. Now they were being asked to implement another model but this time they had administrative, research and medical endorsement.

*Step three* The third step in Lippitt's theory involves assessing the role of the change agent and the initiation of a teaching strategy. The identification of change agents' roles followed Ottoway's (1980) classification of change generator, change implementor and change adopter. The researcher would be the external change agent (change generator) who would carry out the initial teaching and facilitation of the change. In this role he would encourage the development of trust, honesty and a concentration on the objectives of change and the roles of others in reaching these objectives. He always tried to be accessible either in person or by telephone.

It was proposed by the researcher and agreed upon by the staff that there should be internal change agents. Most of the staff were change agents in their own right in that they were involved in the practical decisions on the adoption of the change (change adopters). However, one ward sister took on the role of the primary internal change agent. She was studying for a degree in psychology and welcomed the challenge. The other ward sister became the associate internal change agent taking a more active role when her colleague was off duty. These two managers were well respected by their staff and patients and represented what Ottoway called 'change implementors'. Therefore the change process was to be a collaborative one in which the practitioners themselves were encouraged to accept the locus of control for the change and to take ownership of it.

In early September 1989 formal and informal teaching sessions took place over a two week period and were held on the ward. The researcher discussed with the staff what models were, their advantages and disadvantages and how they can be used in practice. At no stage was it taught that models were the answer to all their problems. Rather they were presented as tools that nurses could use to care for patients. It was pointed out that like all tools models can be useful or useless depending on the situation.

The HNM was explained and discussed with the staff. To involve them actively in the teaching sessions the Minshull et al (1986) article, which describes the HNM, was given to the staff and they were able to apply it to hypothetical patient care situations. They were then asked to help design documentation for its introduction. The result of these discussions was a five page assessment document and care plan specific to the application of the HNM in Ward X. It was stressed that the model's philosophy must be reflected in the care carried out with patients not just in the documentation. Senior nurse management agreed to meet the printing costs when the final draft had been agreed.

Due to their heavy workload and unfamiliarity with the HNM, tutors from the college of nursing were not involved in the teaching sessions. However several informal meetings were held with the clinical teacher, nurse tutor and senior nurse tutor responsible for students' supervision in long-stay care. They were happy that the students were benefiting educationally by being part of a research study and from seeing a different nursing model being implemented.

*Step four* Step four of Lippitt's theory involved the actual implementation of the HNM. Realistic objectives were set as to the pace of its introduction. Further, a common understanding was gained on what was to be done, who was to do what, how it was to be done and when it was to be done. As a pilot exercise the staff selected two 'good' patients and with their permission the HNM was applied to their care.

Although the teaching sessions had been useful in describing the model it was only through using it that the staff began to learn the necessary implementation skills. Throughout this pilot exercise they came together regularly for mutual support, informal teaching and for discussions on the practical problems that arose. These sessions were valuable for standardising the implementation approach and for making the model more meaningful for them. The meetings also helped to minimize their fears and anxieties about the change.

Results from the pilot exercise led to some adaptations in how the model was later implemented. Alongside Orem's assessment sheet the staff had previously used a blank page to record a synopsis of the patient's history. This gave new staff and students an insight into the patient's past. It was decided to retain this as part of the HNM documentation.

The staff also decided to stop identifying patients' needs that cannot be met. With Orem's model (1980) they had identified as many as twelve problems for some patients. Looking back through records it appeared that these were perennial problems that were never solved. For example, the following problem was in one patient's care plan for over a year: "refuses to take part in groupwork." This woman was nearly eighty years of age and although very sociable she preferred not to sit in on discussion groups. It was suggested that a more realistic assessment should be directed at identifying those patient's needs that the nurse is able to meet with particular emphasis on what the patient and their family see as the need. When the model was finally used with all patients this decision meant that most had no more than five problems identified at any time with two patients having no problems at all.

Gradually other staff wished to use the model with their patients and with the support of the ward nursing team this was achieved. For a short time the old documentation based upon Orem's model was completed alongside the new documentation. This obviously led to extra work but it was done in case the change to the new model was unsuccessful. However, when the care of ten patients (n = 18) had changed to the HNM, the old documentation was consigned to the bottom drawer of the filing cabinet. By the end of October 1989 the care of all patients on Ward X was being planned, carried out and evaluated based upon the HNM.

Because of its large psychosocial emphasis, the HNM helped nurses to identify more psychosocial problems than had previously been the case. This led to an increasing role for the two nurses from the social therapy department who were able to use individual and group exercises based upon the problems identified in the care plan. For example assertiveness groups and self awareness groups were organized for small numbers of patients. The ward staff also became more involved in individual and group therapeutic activities.

*Step five* The fifth step in Lippitt's theory involves consolidating the change agents' roles. In August and September 1989 the external change agent was spending between five and six days per week on the research wards. By mid November this was consciously reduced to between three and four days per week. This reflected a gradual movement away from a change generating role to a more consultative role. As internal change agents, the two ward sisters were becoming adept at using the model and as a result they expanded their role as promoters and coordinators of the change. Although the nursing officer visited both research wards regularly his role in the change process was one of enabler and supporter rather than one of active involvement.

*Step six* Step six in Lippitt's theory of planned change concerns the maintenance of the change and its integration into the values and behaviours of the organizational members. Essentially this meant that the momentum of the change was maintained and old practices were not reestablished. This was achieved by having regular consolidation meetings with the staff to discuss progress, to support each other with problems and to remotivate those staff who may be prematurely taking the change for granted.

Initially these meetings took place in the late evening once every week. This was to ensure that the night staff were able to attend. However although the night staff contributed to discussions on issues such as the patients' need for sleeping, a safe environment and evening social diversions they tended to take a less active role then the day staff. This may have been because there were only four of them, two of whom were enrolled nurses.

Perhaps the most common matter discussed at these consolidation meetings was whether each practitioner had as a 'mind set' the philosophy of the model while they were caring for patients. Everyone was aware that if the momentum of change was not maintained the HNM could become a paper exercise. There was always a period of frustration when new students replaced those who were familiar with the change.

170

Whenever possible they were allocated to a key worker, who with the ward sisters, taught them the necessary knowledge and skills required to use the HNM. It normally took students a fortnight to become adept at using it with patients.

In December the primary internal change agent was offered promotion. She took up her new position early in the new year. As the senior ward sister on Ward X she had played a major role in implementing the change. It was initially felt by the researcher that her leaving would jeopardize the project. This feeling was based upon the research of Alexander and Orton (1988) and Miller (1989) who had stressed the importance of the ward sister role in implementing change. Furthermore, could it be possible that five months into the study the use of the HNM had an effect on the dependent variables? Could it also be possible that the departure of the main internal change agent was going to negate any such effect? These questions could only be answered with the aid of an interim post-test.

The researcher was faced with a methodological dilemma; if the primary internal change agent left her 'mortality' could be a threat to the internal validity of the study. Yet if an extra post-test was undertaken the subjects could get bored or over familiar with the research instruments. This 'testing' factor was also a threat to internal validity. However since there would be at least three months before the final post-test a decision was made to undertake an interim post-test (post-test 1) in mid December 1989. Patients and Staff were involved in this decision.

The data for post-test 1 were collected in as similar way as possible to that of the pre-test four months earlier. A letter was sent to each patient and staff member asking them for their assistance in this regard. Yet the data collection process was not without its problems. Unfortunately the external assessors were on annual leave and so the AAI was not used in post-test 1. Moreover Christmas time is not an ideal occasion to undertake data collection. In the days leading up to Christmas patients were going to parties and concerts, there were many visits from voluntary bodies, staff were engaged in organising entertainment, decorating the wards and concentrating on their own extra-mural parties. Despite these obstacles the data were collected from the environment and from patients before Christmas and the staff began to return their postal questionnaires in early January.

After Christmas, as part of hospital policy, one of the ward managers was moved from Ward Y. This meant that there was only one ward manager on each research ward. On Ward X the remaining ward sister took on the role of the main internal change agent.

On Ward X in the first two months of 1990 unforeseen problems occurred that

171

threatened to have consequences for the successful progress of the study. In January an influenza epidemic had an effect on hospital staffing levels. The nursing officer had to move staff for short periods from both wards to build up the complement on acute and psychogeriatric areas. He developed a rota system so that the absences were short and were rotated among the staff. Moreover, he tried to keep the staffing levels on Ward X and Y as similar as possible even when this meant only three staff on each ward. The epidemic also caused a temporary increase in the number of physical and medical problems appearing in the patients' care plans.

In February 1990 a rumour began to circulate around the research wards that they would soon be faced with closure. Apple villa was to become an administrative block and the patients in Ward X and Ward Y were to be moved to other wards. Enquiries suggested that the rumour was false but many patients were visibly worried. This was the topic of conversation for almost two weeks and caused apathy among staff and patients alike. However the rumour was soon forgotten and things returned to normal.

The remaining six weeks of the planned change were spent consolidating the HNM's position on Ward X. In the early part of the change process the subjects were reliant on the external change agent for knowledge, support and guidance. Now, in the latter part of the change, he was only spending about one or two days every week in the hospital. The internal change agent had taken control for coordinating the change and for preventing discontinuance. She was also guiding the change more and more towards practitioner and patient ownership and towards terminating the relationship with the external change agent.

*Post-intervention*

*Step seven* Step seven of Lippitt's theory concerns the termination of the change relationship. After March 1990 the HNM was an accepted part of patient care on Ward X. The data for Post-test2 were collected in the same manner as was described in the pre-test. A letter was sent to each subject pointing out that this was the final collection of information and thanking them for their participation in the study. The external assessors were able to collect data for the AAI.

In the first week of April 1990 the researcher had separate meetings with the subjects (staff and patients) on Ward X and Ward Y. It was evident from the discussions with those on the former ward that the stability of the HNM was no longer dependent on the researcher's presence. The researcher withdrew from the research setting.

172

## Data analysis plan

It is proposed to analyse the raw data using the personal computer version of SPSS (Norusis, 1988). This was done to see if the HNM had any effect on the specified quality of care indicators.

There is much debate among statisticians as to the suitability of parametric and non-parametric tests for different types of data. Knapp (1990) and Bryman and Crammer (1990) attempt to resolve the controversy. They suggest that parametric tests are used if the samples are large, if the data are at the interval or ratio level, are normally distributed and have equal variances. Within the present study most of the research instruments are composed of ordinal scales. Furthermore the samples are small and the data cannot be assumed to be normally distributed or have equal variances. Therefore the inferential statistical tests of choice are nonparametric.

The difference between pre-test and post-test scores (change scores) were calculated on each ward. In order to detect if there are any differences in change scores between Ward X and Ward Y the Mann Whitney U test for independent samples will be applied to the data. It is also proposed to check for statistically significant differences between pre-test and post-test scores on each research ward. The non-parametric statistical test for this type of related data is the Wilcoxon matched pairs sign rank test (Siegal and Castellan, 1988).

The significance levels (alpha level) will be set at $P < 0.05$ for the Mann-Whitney tests. This will be regarded as the minimal acceptable level for statistical significance. There is, however, the possibility that the use of a large number of statistical tests will result in some significant results because of the law of averages. For instance for each ward the Wilcoxon test will be carried out to compare the scores between pre-test and post-test1, between pre-test and post-test2 and between post-test1 and post-test2. Therefore a significance level of 0.02 will be used with this test $(0.05/3 = 0.016)$. The median scores for each dependent variable will be presented in tables and histograms. The reason for using the median instead of the mean as a measure of central tendency was based on the ordinal nature of the data.

# 12 Presentation of findings

In this chapter it is proposed to present the findings around Donabedian's quality of care components - Structure, Process and Outcome. There were three distinct data collection points (pre-test, post-test1 and post-test2). For ease of reference the relevant null and alternative hypotheses highlighted in Chapter twelve are restated here.

$H^0a$ Change scores in the dependent variables are identical between Ward X and Ward Y over the research period.

$H^1a$ Change scores in the dependent variables will be larger in a positive direction in Ward X compared to Ward Y.

$H^0b$ There will be no change in dependent variable scores on Ward X or Ward Y between the three data collection points.

$H^1b$ Post-test scores for the dependent variables on Ward X will be larger in a positive direction than pre-test scores.

The ability or inability to reject the null hypotheses are reported based on the results obtained from the Mann Whitney U test and the Wilcoxon test respectively. These presentations are supported by pertinent descriptive statistics.

## Measurement of structure

*Psychiatric ward monitor*

Ward monitor is an integral part of psychiatric monitor. Its content focuses mainly

174

on the structure of a long-stay psychiatric ward. It is composed of ninety four items and this number represents the highest possible ward monitor score. Results for Ward X and Ward Y over the three data collection points are presented in figure 12.1.

**Figure 12.1. Histogram of ward monitor scores on both Ward X and Ward Y for the three data collection periods**

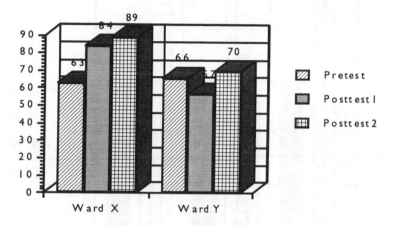

Figure 12.1 shows that although Ward Y had a marginally better pre-test ward monitor score, Ward X increased its pre-test score by twenty six points at post-test2. In contrast Ward Y, after a nine point decrease at post-test1, only increased its post-test2 score by four points from its pre-test position. Therefore at both post-tests the score for Ward X increased while the score for Ward Y decreased.

*Patients and staff ward atmosphere scale scores*

As outlined in the previous chapter there are two WAS instruments. The 'real' WAS gives respondents the opportunity to indicate their perception of the actual atmosphere on their ward. The 'ideal' WAS enables them to indicate what the ward atmosphere should ideally be like. Both instruments were used with patients and staff on Ward X and Ward Y over the research period. The WAS may be sub divided into three dimensions: Relationships (Dim 1 - maximum score 12); Personal Development (Dim 2 - maximum score 16); and Administrative Structure (Dim 3 - maximum score 12). The distribution of patients' median scores for each of these dimensions by ward and by test are shown in figure 12.2.

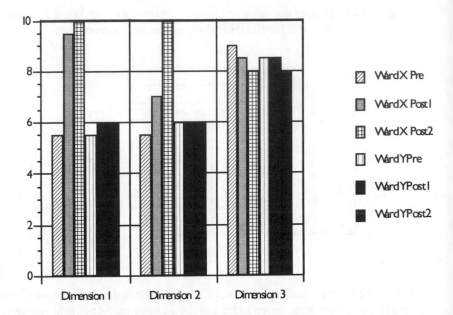

Figure 12.2 shows that for the dimension Relationship (Dim 1) the pre-test patients'
scores on Ward X and Ward Y were similar. Ward X improved over the first and
second post-tests. Ward Y also improved over the same period but very much less.
For the dimension Personal Development (Dim 2) the pre-test patient scores were
lower on Ward X compared to Ward Y. However on the former there was
improvement over the first and second post-tests whereas on the latter there was little
change. For the dimension Administrative Structure (Dim 3) the scores decreased
on both wards with Ward X having a marginally larger decline.

On both wards the patients' and staffs' perception of the ideal ward atmosphere was
obtained so that it could be estimated if their 'real' score got closer to their 'ideal' score
over the research period. The scores for the three dimensions were combined to form
a total WAS score. The distribution of total real scores with ideal scores for patients
is shown in figure 12.3.

**Figure 12.3. Total WAS 'Real' and 'Ideal' scores for patients on Ward X and Ward Y over the research period**

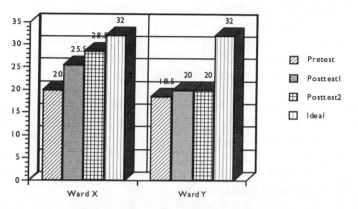

Figure 12.3 shows that patients' perceptions of the ideal ward atmosphere was similar on both wards. However, taking the WAS as a whole, the total pre-test score for patients on Ward X was better than for those on Ward Y. Moreover, for the pre-test to post-test2 period the score for patients on Ward X improved towards the ideal score while patients on Ward Y had only a slight improvement. Therefore while the Real WAS scores on Ward X approached the Ideal scores the Real scores on Ward Y progressed in this direction hardly at all.

The results of how nursing staff on each ward responded to the three WAS dimensions are presented in figure 12.4.

**Figure 12.4. Staff WAS median scores for each WAS dimension on Ward X and Ward Y over the research period**

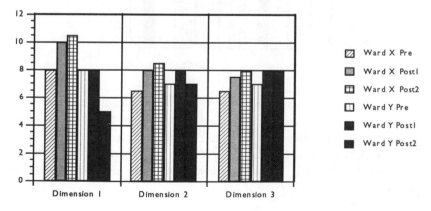

Figure 12.4 shows that the pre-test staff scores for the Relationship dimension (Dim 1) were similar on Ward X and Ward Y. In the former there was improvement over the first and second post-tests whereas in the latter there was no change at post-test1 and disimprovement at post-test2. The staff scores from the Personal Development dimension (Dim 2) indicate that the pre-test results for Ward X were lower than those on Ward Y. However scores on Ward X improved at post-test1 and again at post-test2 while there was little improvement on Ward Y.

The frequency data collected show that the staffs' pre-test scores for the Administrative Structure dimension (Dim 3) were also lower on Ward X than on Ward Y. However the score for the former ward showed a gradual improvement over the research period while on the latter ward the score improved at post-test1 but showed little difference after that. Figure 12.5 shows the distribution of total real WAS scores with ideal scores for staff on Ward X and Ward Y.

**Figure 12.5. Total WAS median 'Real' and 'Ideal' scores for staff on Ward X and Ward Y over the research period**

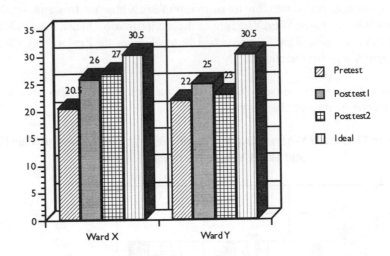

The total WAS scores show that staff on Ward Y had a better pre-test result and both wards improved their score at post-test1. However at post-test2 the score on Ward X had continued to improve while Ward Y's score deceased. Therefore while the staffs' WAS 'Real' score on Ward X approached their perception of their 'Ideal' score, the 'Real' score on Ward Y improved little in this direction over the same period.

To see if there was a significant difference in the amount of change in WAS scores on Ward X compared to Ward Y the Mann-Whitney U test was applied to the change scores. Results are presented in table 12.1.

**Table 12.1.  Mann-Whitney U results comparing how staff and patients' changed their WAS scores over the study period**

|  | staff's WAS | patients' WAS |
|---|---|---|
| PRE-TEST |  |  |
| (Aug, 89) | 60.5 .3173 (ns) | 76.0 .3512 (ns) |
|  | (2 tailed test) |  |
|  |  |  |
| POST-TEST1 |  |  |
| (Xmas, 89) | 29.5 .0066 (*) | 26.5 .0007 (*) |
|  | (1 tailed test) |  |
|  |  |  |
| POST-TEST2 |  |  |
| (April, 90) | 36.0 .0220 (*) | 22.5 .0003 (*) |
|  | (1 tailed test) |  |

(ns = non significant; * significant at 5% alpha)

The Mann-Whitney results in table 12.1 show that there were no significant differences between Ward X and Ward Y at pre-test. This result was the same regardless whether the perceptions were from staff or patients. However when the amount of change in WAS scores was compared at both post-tests staff and patients on Ward X had significantly higher scores compared to those on Ward Y. Therefore at post-test1 and post-test2 the null hypothesis ($H^0a$) was rejected and the alternative hypothesis was accepted ($H^1a$).

To see if the total WAS scores on either Ward X or Ward Y changed significantly over the research period the Wilcoxon matched pairs signed rank test was applied to the staff and patient data. The results are presented in table 12.2.

179

## Table 12.2. Wilcoxon results of WAS scores for patients and staff on Ward X and Ward Y over the study period

|  | WARD X<br>1 tailed test | WARD Y<br>2 tailed test |
|---|---|---|
| Patients' total WAS score |  |  |
| PRE-TEST to POST-TEST1 | 3.5162 (*) | 2.4006 (ns) |
| PRE-TEST to POST-TEST2 | 3.5162 (*) | 2.1783 (ns) |
| POST-TEST1 to POST-TEST2 | 0.0000 (*) | 0.5920 (ns) |
| staffs' total WAS score |  |  |
| PRE-TEST to POST-TEST1 | 2.8633 (*) | 1.0502 (ns) |
| PRE-TEST to POST-TEST2 | 2.6229 (*) | 0.1529 (ns) |
| POST-TEST1 to POST-TEST2 | 1.5289 (ns) | 1.3624 (ns) |

(ns = non significant; * significant at 2% alpha)

From table 12.2 results from the Wilcoxon test indicate that for staff and patients on Ward Y there was no significant change in WAS scores between the three data collection points. Therefore for these WAS scores there was not enough evidence to reject the null hypothesis. In contrast there was a significant change in WAS scores for staff and patients on Ward X. This change was in a positive direction and significant at the 2% alpha level. The exception to this was the change from post-test1 to post-test2 which was not significant at the specified level. Despite this, the null hypothesis ($H^0b$) was rejected and the alternative hypothesis ($H^1b$) was accepted.

The results of the Armitage assessment instrument (AAI) scored by two external assessors are presented in figure 12.6. The highest possible score that could be achieved for each application of the scale was two hundred and thirty one points

**Figure 12.6. External assessors' AAI scores for Ward X and Ward Y at pre-test and post-test2**

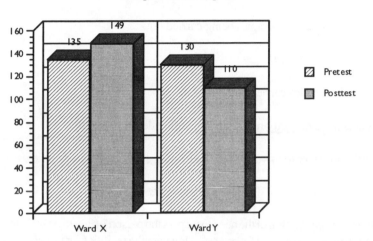

The data illustrated in figure 12.6 represents the average AAI score of each external assessor. For reasons previously explained there were no post-test1 data. Figure 12.6 indicates that the post-test2 scores on the AAI increased on Ward X but decreased on Ward Y.

Each assessor was also able to make comments on aspects of quality on Ward X and on Ward Y. It must be remembered that neither assessor was told what the independent variable was nor which ward was the experimental or control. Furthermore, to avoid any contrived changes to the ward structure between data collection points no one other than the researcher had access to the external assessors' pre-test findings.

*Ward X - external assessors' pre-test comments*

> The arrangement of chairs in the day room is in the form of a 'horse shoe' This does not facilitate patient to patient interaction. The chairs form a partition in the day room.
>
> Privacy was not very evident for patients or relatives.

Decor poor - the ward could do with painting. (It has been brought to my attention that both wards are to be painted soon).

Bed area cold on arrival due to a lot of windows being open.

Care plans seem to be very ritualistic. The problems are mostly medically and physically orientated and although they told me that they use 'Orem' - I see little evidence of it!

Little evidence of therapies being carried out.

No untidiness noted.

No real therapies carried out on Ward.

Seems to be minority rule (staff) regarding decision making.

Television very loud - patients not encouraged to learn new hobbies.

*Ward X - external assessors' post-test2 comments*

There is a recognition of the need to respect the person's right to be self directing and an increased respect for privacy. However the facilities for privacy are poor. The visitors' room is very small. But at least the staff recognize this. There is an awareness of and action against institutional factors.

There is a recognition of the importance of keeping patients up to date on current affairs and hobbies such as knitting and games such as bingo and cards are encouraged.

The care plans are realistic and for two patients there are no problems at all. This appears appropriate for their particular needs. Patients seem to be involved in care planning and the plan is being implemented with them not on them.

Care appears more patient centred and individualistic.

The overall atmosphere is positive rather than repressive. There is a feeling of worth and progression on the ward.

There seems to be a trend to let patients buy their own clothes in town as opposed to wearing hospital clothes.

While talking to a few patients they clearly saw the ward as their home and would be reluctant to leave it.

The decor has improved beyond recognition since my last visit.

The staff appear proud of the ward. It does have the atmosphere of a home in the real sense of the word.

There are several therapeutic groups run by nurses, nurses from social therapy, ward nurses and by student nurses under supervision.

*Ward Y - external assessors' Pre-test comments*

There does not appear to be any real opportunities for privacy for the men themselves nor for their visitors.

The 'therapies' are relinquished to OT staff.

Nursing staff appear to be more concerned with hygiene and less structured occupations. Ward is tidy but paintwork is poor.

Institutionalization very marked.

Care plans are reminiscent of old kardex system - seem to be used for assessment only - plenty of information on the office notice board about Orem's model but this is not reflected in the care plan.

Ward routines and ward norms have a great importance.

Some staff sitting around the television set - patients sitting round the walls.

*Ward Y - external assessors' post-test2 comments*

The ward has been painted and the decor is very pleasing to the eye. However the 'old bathroom' where some patients congregate, although newly decorated, is very cold and impersonal. Most patients enter and leave the ward through here.

Patients sit around the walls of the day room. The semi-circle of chairs around the television is occupied by two students and one staff member (reading a paper). The staff member was still sitting there as I left the ward.

Ward routine and ritual are a template for practice.

The assessment part of the care plans is better than any other part - room for improvement though.

Student nurses seem bored and when questioned they said that they were 'enjoying the break'. They appear to be 'marking time'. No obvious therapies carried out on the ward.

This ward reminds me of an institutionalized hostel for long-stay patients - this ward, to an outsider, could not be considered to be the patients' home.

## Measures of process

*Psychiatric patients' monitor*

The psychiatric patient monitor is constructed around the processes of care. It is composed of seventy five items divided into three subscales: Care Planning, Meeting Physical Needs and Meeting Psychosocial Needs. Median scores for each of these subscales are presented in figure 12.7.

**Figure 12.7. Median scores for patient monitor subscales on Ward X and Ward Y over the research period**

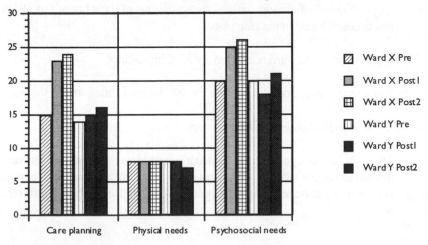

Figure 12.7 shows that for the subscale Care Planning the scores on Ward X improved over both post-tests, while on Ward Y the improvement was much less. For the subscale Meeting Physical Needs Ward X's score did not change over the entire research period, whereas on Ward Y there was no change in score at the first Post-test and a disimprovement at the second. Similarly Ward X improved on the subscale Meeting Psychosocial Needs at post-test1 and post-test2 while on Ward Y there was decrease in score at the first Post-test but improvement at the second. The total patient monitor score for both wards over the research period is presented in figure 12.8.

**Figure 12.8. Median scores for total patient monitor scores on Ward X and Ward Y over the research period**

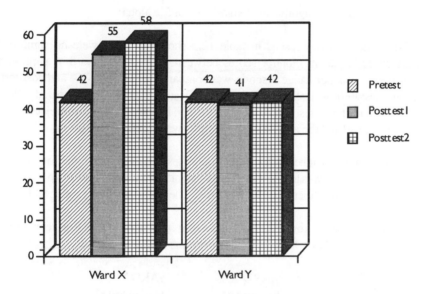

From figure 12.8 it can be observed that the total patient monitor scores for Ward X show an improvement over both post-tests. On Ward Y however, there was a slight decrease at post-test1 and a return to pre-test levels at post-test2. Viewed as a percentage increase over the entire research period, Ward Y improved by one percent while Ward X improved by twenty four percent.

The Mann-Whitney U test was applied to the total patient monitor change scores. This was undertaken to see if there was a more positive change in the care given on Ward X compared to Ward Y over the research period. Results are presented in table 12.3.

**Table 12.3. Mann-Whitney U results of total patient monitor change scores between Ward X and Ward Y**

| | |
|---|---|
| PRE-TEST | 80.0 .4780 (ns) |
| (Aug, 89) | (2 tailed test) |
| | |
| POST-TEST1 | 2.05 .0011 (*) |
| (Xmas, 89) | (1 tailed test) |
| | |
| POST-TEST2 | 51.5 .0186 (*) |
| (April, 90) | (1 tailed test) |

(ns = non significant; * significant at 5% alpha)

The Mann-Whitney results in table 12.3 show that there were no significant differences in patient monitor scores between Ward X and Ward Y at pre-test. However, when the change in scores was compared between pre-test and post-test1 and pre-test and post-test2 Ward X had a significantly higher score compared to Ward Y. Therefore at post-test1 and post-test2 the null hypothesis ($H^0a$) was rejected at to 5% alpha level and the alternative hypothesis was accepted ($H^1a$).

The Wilcoxon matched pairs signed ranks test was applied to the total patient monitor data. This was to see if there was a significant change between pre-test and post-test results on either Ward X or Ward Y. The results are presented in table 12.4.

**Table 12.4. Wilcoxon test results showing total patient monitor scores on Ward X and Ward Y over the research period**

| | WARD X<br>1 tailed test | WARD Y<br>2 tailed test |
|---|---|---|
| PRE-TEST to<br>POST-TEST1 | 3.0954 (*) | 0.5491 (ns) |
| PRE-TEST to<br>POST-TEST2 | 3.1801 (*) | 1.4513 (ns) |
| POST-TEST1 to<br>POST-TEST2 | 1.8175 (ns) | 1.4120 (ns) |

(ns = non significant; * significant at 2% alpha)

From table 12.4 the Wilcoxon results indicate that on Ward Y there was no significant change in patient monitor scores between pre-test and both post-tests. Therefore there was a lack of sufficient evidence to reject the null hypothesis ($H^0b$) for Ward Y's results. On Ward X however, there was a significantly higher score when pre-test scores were compared with post-test scores. The exception to this was the post-test1 to post-test2 result which was not significant at the 2% alpha level. Nevertheless overall results still enabled the null hypothesis ($H^0b$) to be rejected and the alternative hypothesis ($H^1b$) to be accepted. When the Wilcoxon and Mann-Whitney U tests are applied to the subscales results they indicate statistically significant improvements on Ward X for Care Planning and Meeting Psychosocial Needs.

*Care plan goals*

Data on the number and type of care plan goals for both Ward X and Ward Y are presented in table 12.5.

**Table 12.5. Number of care plan goals on Ward X and Ward Y by type over the three data collection points**

| GOAL | PRETEST | POST-TEST1 | POST-TEST2 |
|------|---------|------------|------------|
| **WARD X** | | | |
| Physical | 28 | 17 | 19 |
| Psychological | 17 | 11 | 12 |
| Social | 5 | 1 | 1 |
| Medical | 20 | 3 | 1 |
| Cognitive | 0 | 0 | 1 |
| Safety | 1 | 5 | 2 |
| **WARD Y** | | | |
| Physical | 11 | 12 | 10 |
| Psychological | 10 | 8 | 6 |
| Social | 6 | 5 | 5 |
| Medical | 7 | 7 | 5 |
| Cognitive | 5 | 6 | 4 |
| Safety | 0 | 1 | 1 |

Table 12.5 indicates that on Ward X the total number of physical, psychological, social and medical goals decreased over the research period while there was a small increase in the total number of cognitive and safety goals. On Ward Y the overall number of goals was less than that on Ward X and only safety goals increased in number over the research period.

The following comments relate to the content of the goals within the care plans on both wards. On Ward X the pre-test goals tended to be:

1.    long range time frame such as two months or more in some cases;
2.    nurse-centred rather than patient-centred;
3.    long winded - having two or three goals in each goal;
4.    medically oriented;
5.    in order of priority medical type goals came first;
6.    were cure centred; for example, 'eliminate cause of pain' 'make patient free from fits';
7.    each patient had five or six (some seven) goals each;
8.    ambiguous; for example, 'reduce weight', 'return to normal';
9.    excessive use of the term 'to reduce...'.

On Ward X post-test1 goals were:

1.    more short range, 1 month being the longest time span;
2.    patient-centred rather than nurse-centred;
3.    showed evidence of using measurement scales;
4.    reduction in the number of goals.

In post-test2 goals on Ward X had benefits of post-test1 factors plus they were:

1.    dated;
2.    used patients name;
3.    were more measurable;
4.    had psychosocial priority unless physical problems were more urgent;
5.    more precise;
6.    less long winded;
7.    tended to have only one major component per goal.

At pre-test the care plans goals on Ward Y showed many similarities to the pre-test goals on Ward X. There were also:

1.    in order of priority physical type goals came first;

188

2. excessive use of the term 'to improve and maintain';
3. some were not goals at all but interventions; for example, 'monitor dress constantly';
4. very broad; for example, 'de-institutionalize'!

In post-test1 care plan goals on Ward Y were invariably the same as pretest goals. In post-test2 a few goals showed evidence of being patient centred in that the patient's name was mentioned in the goal statement. But for most of the care plans the goals were just a repeat of those set nine months previously. The following example from Ward Y showed a worrying trend. In August 1989 a goal 'find cause of left lumbar mass and treat' was still in the careplan in December 1989 and in April 1990 it was still there but with: 'allow necessary treatment to commence as soon as possible'.

## Measures of outcome

*Patient satisfaction*

The patient satisfaction questionnaire is a twenty three item instrument which forms part of psychiatric monitor. The questionnaire is divided into five subscales. The maximum scores for each subscale are indicated in brackets. The subscales are Patient Wellbeing (16); Information Given (24); Physical Care (20); Treatments (12); and Ward Staffing (20). The median scores from the patients on Ward X and Ward Y are presented in figure 12.9.

**Figure 12.9. Patient satisfaction subscale scores (median) for Ward X and Ward Y over the study period**

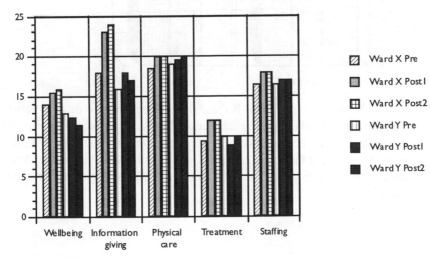

189

Figure 12.9 shows that at post-test1 and post-test2 there was an improvement on all five subscales for patients in Ward X. For patients in Ward Y the Wellbeing score decreased over both post-tests while the subscales Information Given, Physical Care and Staffing improved slightly. Also on Ward Y there was a lowering of score for the subscale Treatment at post-test1 but at post-test2 the scores returned to their pre-test level.

Taking the patient satisfaction questionnaire as a whole each patient could score a maximum of ninety two points or a minimum of twenty three points. Figure 12.10 shows the median scores attained by patients on both wards over the pre-test and post-test data collection points.

**Figure 12.10. Total patient satisfaction scores (median) on Ward X and Ward Y over the three data collection points**

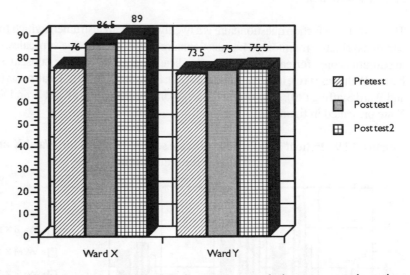

Figure 12.10 shows that on Ward X there was a steady improvement in patient satisfaction scores over the entire research period. On Ward Y an initial improvement in satisfaction scores at post-test1 slowed to an almost imperceptible improvement at post-test2. To see if the score on Ward X were significantly higher the Mann-Whitney U test was applied to the change scores on both wards. Results are presented in table 12.6.

**Table 12.6. Mann-Whitney U results for patient satisfaction change scores between Ward X and Ward Y**

| PRE-TEST | 80.0 .4780 (ns) |
| (Aug, 89) | (2 tailed test) |
| | |
| POST-TEST1 | 36.5 .0022 (*) |
| (Xmas, 89) | (1 tailed test) |
| | |
| POST-TEST2 | 32.0 .0011 (*) |
| (April, 90) | (1 tailed test) |

(ns = non significant; * significant at 5% alpha)

The Mann-Whitney results in table 12.6 show that there were no significant differences in patient satisfaction scores between Ward X and Ward Y at pre-test. However when the change in scores was compared between pre-test and post-test1 and pre-test and post-test2 Ward X had a significantly higher score compared to Ward Y. Therefore at post-test1 and post-test2 the null hypothesis ($H^0a$) was rejected at the 5% alpha level and the alternative hypothesis was accepted ($H^1a$).

The Wilcoxon matched pairs signed rank test was applied to the data to see if a significant change in patient satisfaction scores occurred on either ward over the research period. The results are presented in table 12.7.

**Table 12.7. Wilcoxon test results for patient satisfaction scores on Ward X and Ward Y over the research period**

| | WARD X | WARD Y |
|---|---|---|
| | (1 tailed test) | (2 tailed test) |
| PRE-TEST to POST-TEST1 | 3.4645 (*) | 0.8664 (ns) |
| | | |
| PRE-TEST to POST-TEST2 | 3.5162 (*) | 1.0198 (ns) |
| | | |
| POST-TEST1 to POST-TEST2 | 2.3786 (*) | 0.5883 (ns) |

(ns = non significant; * significant at 2% alpha)

Table 12.7 shows that a significant change occurred (at the 2% alpha level) in patient satisfaction scores on Ward X between pre-test and post-test1 periods. This change was in a positive direction and extended over the pre-test to post-test2 period. The table also shows that satisfaction levels continued to increase significantly over the post-test1 to post-test2 period. In contrast there was no significant change in patient satisfaction levels on Ward Y over the same periods. Therefore there was not enough evidence to reject the null hypothesis ($H^0b$) for patients on Ward Y. However there was sufficient evidence to reject the null hypothesis ($H^0b$) and accept the alternative hypothesis ($H^1b$) for patients in Ward X.

*Nurse satisfaction*

The nurse satisfaction questionnaire is a thirty one item instrument that also forms part of psychiatric monitor. Although it is divided into the same five subscales as the patient satisfaction questionnaire there are more questions. This affects the maximum possible scores: Patient Wellbeing (28); Information Given to Patients (12); Physical Care of Patients (20); Patients' Treatments (12); and Ward Staffing (52). The median scores for Ward X and Ward Y at each data collection point are presented in figure 12.11.

**Figure 12.11. Nurse satisfaction subscale scores (median) for both Ward X and Ward Y over the study period**

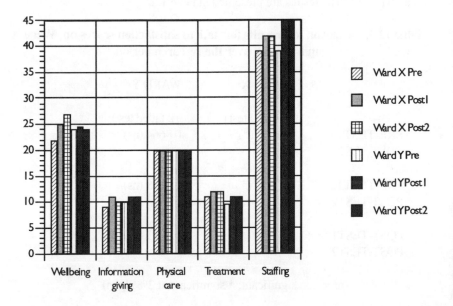

Figure 12.11 shows that nurse satisfaction scores for staff on Ward X improved in all subscales except Physical Care. This subscale retained its pre-test score at both post-tests. On Ward Y the subscale scores for Wellbeing, Information Given and Treatment improved slightly over the research period. The subscale Staffing had the greatest increase in score and the subscale Physical had an identical score pattern to that of Ward X.

The maximum possible score for the complete nurse satisfaction questionnaire is 124 points. Figure 12.12 shows the median satisfaction scores for nursing staff on both wards over the pre-test and post-test data collection points.

**Figure 12.12. Total nurse satisfaction scores (median) on Ward X and Ward Y for the three data collection points**

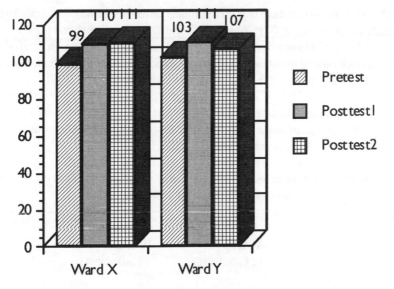

Figure 12.12 shows that on Ward Y the staff had a higher pre-test satisfaction score than those staff on Ward X. This differential persisted at post-test1. However at post-test2 satisfaction levels continued to improve on Ward X while there was a steady decrease in scores on Ward Y.

The Mann-Whitney U test was applied to the change scores to see if during the research period nurse satisfaction results changed significantly on Ward X compared to Ward Y. The results are presented in table 12.8.

**Table 12.8. Mann-Whitney U results for nurse satisfaction change scores between Ward X and Ward Y**

| | | |
|---|---|---|
| PRE-TEST | 80.0 .4780 (ns) | |
| (Aug, 89) | (2 tailed test) | |
| | | |
| POST-TEST1 | 42.0 .1507 (ns) | |
| (Xmas, 89) | (1 tailed test) | |
| | | |
| POST-TEST2 | 49.5 .3164 (ns) | |
| (April, 90) | (1 tailed test) | |

(ns = non significant at 5% alpha)

Table 12.8 shows that there was no significant difference in pre-test scores for nurse satisfaction between staff on Ward X or Ward Y. For post-test1 and post-test2 staff on Ward X did not have a significantly higher change score compared to staff on Ward Y. Therefore taking the nurse satisfaction questionnaire as a whole there was lack of sufficient evidence to reject the null hypothesis ($H^0a$).

The Wilcoxon matched pairs signed ranks test was applied to the data to see if a significant change in nurse satisfaction scores occurred on either ward over the research period. Results are presented in table 12.9.

**Table 12.9. Wilcoxon test results for nurse satisfaction scores on Ward X and Ward Y over the research period**

| | WARD X (1 tailed test) | WARD Y (2 tailed test) |
|---|---|---|
| PRE-TEST to POST-TEST1 | 2.0449 (*) | 1.6082 (ns) |
| PRE-TEST to POST-TEST2 | 1.9560 (*) | 0.9806 (ns) |
| POST-TEST1 to POST-TEST2 | 0.1778 (ns) | 0.8664 (ns) |

(ns = non significant; * significant at 2% alpha)

Table 12.9 shows that nurse satisfaction scores significantly changed (at the 2% alpha level) on Ward X between pre-test and post-test1 periods. This change was in a positive direction and extended over the pre-test to post-test2 period. The change between post-test1 and post-test2 was not statistically significant. Nonetheless the null hypothesis ($H^0b$) was rejected and the alternative hypothesis ($H^1b$) was accepted. During the same period there was no statistically significant change in nurse satisfaction scores on Ward Y. Therefore there was not enough evidence to reject the null hypothesis ($H^0b$) for staff on Ward Y.

*Attitudes towards nursing models*

A 20 item attitude towards nursing models questionnaire was distributed to each member of the nursing staff on both research wards at pre-test, post-test1 and post-test2. Respondents could score a maximum of 100 points. The median scores are presented in figure 12.13.

**Figure 12.13. Attitudes towards models score for staff on Ward X and Ward Y for the three data collection points**

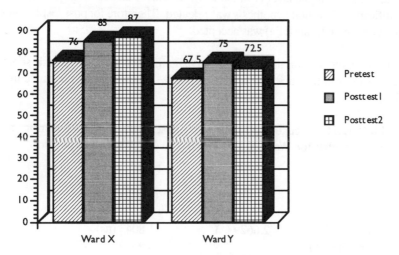

Figure 12.13 indicates that there was an improvement in staffs' attitude towards nursing models on Ward X and Ward Y. However while staff on Ward X improved throughout the research period, staff on Ward Y decreased their score at post-test2.

To see if during the research period the scores on Ward X changed more in a positive direction than on Ward Y the Mann-Whitney U test was applied to the change scores. The results are presented in table 12.10.

**Table 12.10. Mann-Whitney U results for staffs' attitudes towards models score between Ward X and Ward Y**

|  |  |
|---|---|
| PRE-TEST | 80.0 .4780 (ns) |
| (Aug, 89) | (2 tailed test) |
| | |
| POST-TEST1 | 61.0 .3929 (ns) |
| (Xmas, 89) | (1 tailed test) |
| | |
| POST-TEST2 | 33.5 .0439 (*) |
| (Apr, 90) | (1 tailed test) |

(ns = non significant; * significant at 5% alpha)

Table 12.10 shows that at pre-test there was no significant difference between the nursing staff on Ward X and Ward Y concerning their attitudes towards nursing models. The result was the same when change scores were compared at post-test1. Therefore at post-test1 there was not enough evidence to reject the null hypothesis ($H^0a$) at the 5% alpha level (1 tailed test). However the results at post-test2 were significant and the null hypothesis was rejected. Therefore for post-test2 scores the alternative hypothesis ($H^1a$) was accepted.

The Wilcoxon test was used to detect any significant changes in attitude scores on either ward over the three data collection points. The results are presented in table 12.11.

**Table 12.11. Wilcoxon test scores on nurses' attitudes towards nursing models for Ward X and Ward Y over the research period**

|  | WARD X (1 tailed test) | WARD Y (2 tailed test) |
|---|---|---|
| PRE-TEST to POST-TEST1 | 2.6629 (*) | 1.8043 (ns) |
| PRE-TEST to POST-TEST2 | 2.8031 (*) | 0.7060 (ns) |
| POST-TEST1 to POST-TEST2 | 1.1722 (ns) | 1.1255 (ns) |

(ns = non significant; * significant at 2% alpha)

The results in table 12.11 show that on Ward X there was a significant change in nursing staffs' attitudes towards models over the pre-test to post-test1 and pre-test to post-test2 intervals. This change was in a positive direction. Therefore the null hypothesis ($H^0b$) was rejected for both these periods and the alternative hypothesis ($H^1b$) was accepted. However the results for the period post-test1 to post-test2 were non significant at the 2% alpha level. Similarly, results from staff on Ward Y indicate that there was no significant change in their attitudes towards models score over the research period. Therefore for nurses on Ward Y the null hypothesis ($H^0b$) cannot be rejected due to lack of evidence.

*Nurses evaluation of patients' behaviour*

The thirty item nurse observation scale for inpatient evaluation (NOSIE.30) was jointly completed by pairs of nurses on Ward X and Ward Y at the three data collection points. NOSIE 30 may be divided into seven subscales. Some of these are scored positively (Social Competence, Social Interest, Personal Neatness) and some are scored negatively (Irritability, Manifest Psychosis, Retardation, Depression). The median scores for each of these subscales are presented in tables 12.12 and 12.13.

**Table 12.12. Median scores achieved for NOSIE subscales on Ward X at the three data collection points**

|  | PRETEST | POST-TEST1 | POST-TEST2 |
|---|---|---|---|
| Social Competence (best score=20) | 16.0 | 16.0 | 18.0 |
| Social Interest (best score=20) | 8.0 | 10.0 | 12.0 |
| Personal Neatness (best score=16) | 14.0 | 15.0 | 15.0 |
| Irritability (best score=0) | 4.0 | 4.0 | 3.0 |
| Manifest Psychosis (best score=0) | 3.0 | 1.0 | 1.0 |
| Retardation (best score=0) | 4.0 | 5.0 | 5.0 |
| Depression (best score=0) | 3.0 | 2.0 | 1.0 |

**Table 12.13. Median scores achieved for NOSIE subscales on Ward Y at the three data collection points**

| | PRETEST | POST-TEST1 | POST-TEST2 |
|---|---|---|---|
| Social Competence (best score=20) | 15.5 | 17.5 | 17.0 |
| Social Interest (best score=20) | 10.0 | 6.5 | 8.0 |
| Personal Neatness (best score=16) | 12.0 | 11.0 | 11.5 |
| Irritability (best score=0) | 4.0 | 2.5 | 2.5 |
| Manifest Psychosis (best score=0) | 1.0 | 0.5. | 1.0 |
| Retardation (best score=0) | 4.0 | 4.0 | 4.5 |
| Depression (best score=0) | 1.0 | 1.0 | 1.0 |

Tables 12.12 shows that patients on Ward X improved their median scores over the research period on all NOSIE subscales except retardation. Table 12.13 shows that for patients on Ward Y the changes in subscales at post-test1 and post-test2 were more variable. There was a change in a positive direction for Social Competence and Irritability, a disimprovement for Social Interest, Personal Neatness and Retardation and no change for Manifest Psychosis and Depression. To give a complete picture of score changes on both wards total scores were calculated. To do this Honigfeld and Klett (1965) use the following formula: 96 + total positive scores - total negative scores. The total scores for both wards over the research period are presented in figure 12.14.

## Figure 12.14. Total median scores achieved for the NOSIE scale on both Ward X and Ward Y over the research period

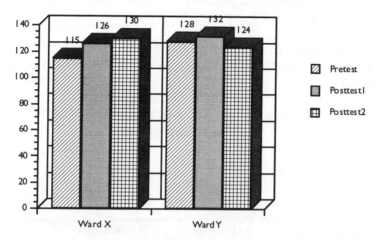

Figure 12.14 indicates that there was an improvement among patients on Ward X over both post-tests. On Ward Y the patients started with a higher NOSIE score and there was an improvement at post-test1. However at post-test2 the scores decreased to a level below their pre-test level.

To detect if these results were statistically different in favour of patients on Ward X the change scores on both wards were compared using the Mann-Whitney U test. Results are shown in table 12.14.

## Table 12.14. Mann-Whitney U results of NOSIE change scores betwee Ward X and Ward Y over the research period

| | | |
|---|---|---|
| PRE-TEST | 78.0 | .3033 (ns) |
| (Aug, 89) | (2 tailed test) | |
| | | |
| POST-TEST1 | 86.5 | .4985 (ns) |
| (Xmas, 89) | (1 tailed test) | |
| | | |
| POST-TEST2 | 68.0 | .1398 (ns) |
| (April, 90) | (1 tailed test) | |

(ns = non significant at 5% alpha)

Table 12.14 shows that there was no significant difference in NOSIE scores between Ward X and Ward Y at pre-test. Further, when the change scores were compared there was no significant difference at post-test1 or post-test2. Therefore there was lack of evidence to reject the null hypothesis ($H^0a$).

To see if the NOSIE scores changed significantly over the research period on either Ward X or Ward Y the Wilcoxon test was applied to the data. Results are presented in table 12.15.

**Table 12.15. Wilcoxon test results for NOSIE scores on Ward X and Ward Y over the research period**

|  | WARD X<br>1 tailed test) | WARD Y<br>(2 tailed test) |
|---|---|---|
| PRE-TEST to<br>POST-TEST1 | 1.1598 (ns) | 0.1400 (ns) |
| PRE-TEST to<br>POST-TEST2 | 2.6746 (*) | 0.3058 (ns) |
| POST-TEST1 to<br>POST-TEST2 | 1.8175 (ns) | 0.0510 (ns) |

(ns = non significant; * significant at 2% alpha)

Table 12.15 shows that on Ward X there was no significant change in NOSIE scores over the pre-test to post-test1 and the post-test1 to post-test2 periods. However there were significant changes between pre-test and post-test2. Therefore for this result there was sufficient evidence to reject the null hypothesis ($H^0b$) and accept the alternative hypothesis ($H^1b$). Since there were no significant changes on Ward Y the null hypothesis ($H^0b$) was not rejected for patients there.

*Patient dependency levels*

The patient dependency scale used within this study was completed as part of psychiatric monitor. Patients could score a maximum of thirty five points or a minimum of ten points. Since a high score suggests a high dependency level, a decrease in dependency score over the research period suggests an improvement. The median scores are depicted in figure 12.15.

**Figure 12.15. Patient dependency scores for patients on Ward X and Ward Y at the three data collection points**

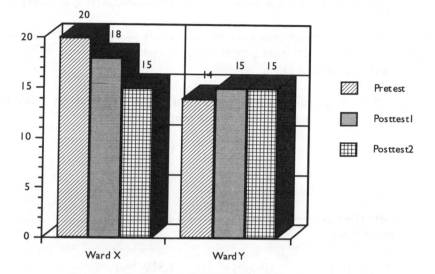

Figure 12.15 shows that patients on Ward X were more dependent at pre-test than patients on Ward Y. However the dependency scores for both post-tests improved on Ward X while they worsened on Ward Y. To note if these results were statistically significant in favour of Ward X the Mann-Whitney U test was applied to the change scores. The results are presented in table 12.16.

**Table 12.16. Mann-Whitney U results for patient dependency change scores on Ward X and Ward Y**

| | |
|---|---|
| PRE-TEST | 36.0 .0012 (*) |
| (Aug, 89) | (2 tailed test) |
| | |
| POST-TEST1 | 26.0 .0002 (*) |
| (Xmas, 89) | (1 tailed test) |
| | |
| POST-TEST2 | 10.5 .0000 (*) |
| (Apr, 90) | (1 tailed test) |

(* significant at 5% alpha)

Table 12.16 shows that there was a significant difference at pre-test between the wards. This was because the base line dependency scores for the patients on Ward

Y were better than for those on Ward X. However at post-test1 and post-test2 Ward X had a greater change in a positive direction than patients on Ward Y. Therefore the null hypothesis ($H^0a$) was rejected and the alternative hypothesis ($H^1a$) was accepted.

To detect if patient dependency scores significantly changed over the research period on either Ward X or Ward Y the Wilcoxon test was applied to the data. Results are presented in table 12.17.

**Table 12.17. Wilcoxon test results for patient dependency levels on Ward X and Ward Y over the research period**

|  | WARD X (1 tailed test) | WARD Y (2 tailed test) |
|---|---|---|
| PRE-TEST to POST-TEST1 | 3.1798 (*) | 2.2014 (ns) |
| PRE-TEST to POST-TEST2 | 3.5162 (*) | 1.5289 (ns) |
| POST-TEST1 to POST-TEST2 | 3.5162 (*) | 0.4890 (ns) |

(ns = non significant; * significant at 2% alpha)

Table 12.17 shows that patient dependency scores on Ward X changed significantly over the entire research period. Therefore for patients on Ward X the null hypothesis ($H^0b$) was rejected and the alternative hypothesis ($H^1b$) was accepted. On Ward Y the change in patient dependency was not significant at the 2% alpha level. Therefore for Ward Y there was not enough evidence to reject the null hypothesis ($H^0b$).

*Medication patterns*

The medication kardexes on Ward X and Ward Y were scrutinized over the research period in order to detect any changes in prescribing patterns. All the drugs used on both wards could be included in the following four categories: Phenothiazines, Anti-depressants, Anti-parkinson and Physical medications (diuretics, cardiac drugs, aperients etc). The number of patients on these medications are shown in table 12.18.

**Table 12.18. Number of patients on Ward X (n=18) and Ward Y (n=14)
being prescribed different medication over the research period**

PRETEST  POST-TEST1  POST-TEST2

WARD X

| | PRETEST | POST-TEST1 | POST-TEST2 |
|---|---|---|---|
| Phenothiazines | 15 | 15 | 15 |
| Anti-depressants | 3 | 3 | 3 |
| Physical medications | 14 | 15 | 14 |
| Anti-parkinson | 6 | 6 | 6 |

WARD Y

| | PRETEST | POST-TEST1 | POST-TEST2 |
|---|---|---|---|
| Phenothiazines | 10 | 10 | 10 |
| Anti-depressants | 0 | 1 | 0 |
| Physical medications | 4 | 3 | 6 |
| Anti-parkinson | 4 | 4 | 4 |

Table 12.18 shows  that  apart from some minor changes in physical and antidepressant medications the prescribing patterns varied little on either ward over the research period. The table also shows that there were more patients on these medications on Ward X than there were on Ward Y.

To detect if this dissimilarity was significant or merely the result of there being more patients on Ward X the Mann-Whitney U test was applied to the data.   Findings indicate that apart from medications for physical problems there was no significant difference in phenothiazine, anti-depressant and anti-parkinson prescribing patterns for patients on either ward. The same trend continued for post-test1.  For post-test2 there were no significant difference between wards in the prescribing of any of the medication groups.  To see if prescribing patterns changed significantly over the three data collection points on either Ward X or Ward Y the Wilcoxon test was applied to the data. Although there were some changes in drug prescriptions on each ward over the research period these changes were not significant at the 2% alpha level.  A comprehensive presentation of these  results can be found in Appendix Y.

*Psychosocial changes*

When evaluating the introduction of any innovation  in a psychiatric setting one of the most important areas to examine is the change in psychosocial functioning of patients.  Most of  the research instruments used had psychosocial components or subscales.

**Table 12.19. The research instruments whose psychosocial components showed a positive change on Ward X over the research period**

| Research Instrument | Psychosocial Subscale/Component |
|---|---|
| Ward atmosphere scale (patients & staff). | Personal development. relationship. |
| Armitage assessment instrument. | Social mixing & relationships. External assessors comments. |
| Patient monitor. | Psychosocial needs. |
| Patient satisfaction questionnaire. | Wellbeing. Treatment. |
| Nurse satisfaction questionnaire. | Wellbeing. Treatment. |
| NOSIE. | All subscales. |
| Patient dependency form. | Social interaction. |

Table 12.19 shows that there was an improvement on Ward X in those research instruments that had psychosocial components. On Ward Y there were marginal improvements in the 'social competence' and 'irritability' subscales of NOSIE, in the psychosocial subscale of patient monitor and in the 'treatment' subscale of the Staff satisfaction questionnaire. However for the rest of the instruments specified in table 12.19 there was a decrease in psychosocial score on Ward Y. This indicates that when both research wards are compared those psychosocial aspects of patient care as measured by the above instruments improved to a greater extent on Ward X than on ward Y.

# 13 Discussion of results

**Interpretation of results**

In this chapter an attempt will be made to discuss and interpret the findings. This will centre on the results obtained for each dependent variable and how these relate to the extant literature. Emphasis will be placed on whether the null hypotheses were rejected or not. However, the researcher is conscious of the danger of going beyond the data. Unlike true experiments cause and effect relationships cannot easily be assumed for quasi-experimental designs. Therefore it is necessary to explore other possible explanations for changes in the dependent variables.

*'Structure' findings*

Three research instruments were used to measure changes in structure *between* and *within* Ward X and Ward Y over the research period. These were: ward monitor; ward atmosphere scale (WAS); and the Armitage assessment instrument (AAI). The results from these instruments would indicate that there was no significant difference between Ward X or Ward Y at pre-test. However over the research period the scores on both wards changed. Pictorially and statistically the results from Ward X showed a greater improvement than those from Ward Y.

The ward monitor findings were supported by an independent group of evaluators (WHSSB, 1990). They used a different psychiatric monitor tool (Goldstone, 1990) that had been tested for reliability and validity in Northern Ireland. Their results also showed that Ward X had a significantly better ward monitor score than Ward Y (WHSSB, 1990).

Findings from the WAS (see Figs 12.2) indicate that patients and staff on Ward X improved their score on all the WAS dimensions except 'Administrative Structure'. This dimension was concerned with the importance of, and the extent to which patients were familiar with and follow, order and routine. Neither patients nor staff gave this dimension much consideration, preferring not to be too restricted by rules and regulations. Armitage (1990) found a similar reluctance when he used the WAS with long-stay psychiatric patients in Wales. Nevertheless, when the changes in WAS were subjected to statistical tests, Ward X had significant results in a positive direction while Ward Y had not.

On Ward X the pre-test findings from the Armitage assessment instrument noted evidence of routine and institutionalization similar to that described by Barton (1959) and Goffman (1961). When they returned at post-test the external assessors found that the care was more patient centred and care plans were being used as more than just assessment schedules. The patients were given greater freedom and nurses were involved in therapeutic groups. The assessors' post-test comments support these trends and indicate that nurses on Ward X were actively using the HNM with patients. The model was not something that was 'office-bound'; it had a pervading influence on the care given. This improvement in care planning due to the introduction of a nursing model supports the views of Fawcett (1990) in the United States and Crouch (1990) in the United Kingdom.

*'Process' findings.*

The application of patient monitor and the examination of the number, type and content of care plan goals were the two methods used to evaluate changes in the 'Process' of care.

The results from patient monitor would indicate that there was no significant difference between Ward X or Ward Y at pre-test. However when the change scores were subjected to statistical tests the results were significant in favour of Ward X. It has also been mentioned above that an independent group of evaluators applied a different psychiatric monitor instrument to the research wards. Their results corroborate the patient monitor findings discussed here (WHSSB, 1990).

Although there was an increase in score on both wards for the subscales care planning and meeting psychosocial needs the increase on Ward X was much greater than on Ward Y. However considering the emphasis patient monitor places on care planning and on meeting psychosocial needs these findings were not surprising. After all, the largest part of the HNM focuses on psychosocial needs and the meeting of these needs would obviously improve with its introduction. As seen from comments made by external assessors in the AAI the pre-test care planning on Ward X was poor.

Therefore it was not inconceivable that the HNM, if used correctly, would lead to improved post-test care planning.

The data collected on the number and type of care plan goals on both wards gave interesting results. If what was argued in the previous paragraph were true it might have been expected that the number of physical and medical goals would decrease in number on Ward X over the research period. Results in table 12.5 showed that this did occur. It might also have been expected that the number of psychological and social goals would increase on Ward X and that the staffs' expectations for the patients on Ward X would have increased leading to more goals of this type. However table 12.5 showed that between pre-test and post-test1 these goals decreased in number. This could convey the impression that the HNM did not make any difference to psychosocial aspects of care and care planning. But such an interpretation was contradicted by the results from other instruments (see table 12.19).

There is, however, a more plausible explanation for this unexpected finding. Many psychological and social goals noted at pre-test were unrealistic and inappropriate. With the use of the HNM these were subsequently removed. Therefore, although the number of psychosocial goals on Ward X was reduced at Post-test they were more realistic and more patient centred. This general improvement in psychosocial focus on Ward X will be discussed further in the implications section of this report.

Table 12.5 also indicated a lack of cognitive goals in the care plans on Ward X. But patient teaching was taking place there, both within groups and individually. However these interactions tended to be written within the care plan as nursing interventions while on Ward Y they were written as goals (for example, 'educate him re his condition'). This explains the high profile given to cognitive goals within the care plans of Ward Y.

Therefore the quality of the care plan goals on Ward X improved over the research period while Ward Y varied little over the same period. This supports the findings from the AAI and the results from the care planning subscale within patient monitor. It also lends support to the writings of Meleis (1985) on the positive effects of nursing models on goal identification.

*'Outcome' findings.*

In this study, six measures were employed to evaluate the effects of the HNM on outcomes. Four were patient orientated: patient satisfaction, NOSIE, medication patterns and patient dependency. Two were staff orientated: staff satisfaction and attitudes towards nursing models.

Results presented in figure 12.10 showed that patient satisfaction improved on both Ward X and Ward Y. This finding is supportive of American research which suggests that because of fear of staff retaliation, a desire to please, a fear of being ungrateful or because of the 'halo effect' patients seldom wish to appear dissatisfied (Ventura et al, 1982; LaMonica et al, 1986). This tendency towards satisfaction has also been seen among psychiatric patients in British studies (Raphael, 1972; Barker, 1988; Armitage, 1990).

However this does not explain the significantly greater increase in patient satisfaction on Ward X. Most of the events extraneous to the study that could be influential would have also affected the patients on Ward Y. Other studies on the use of nursing models have found similar significant improvements in patient satisfaction levels (Hoch, 1987; Kemp, 1990).

Most of the nurse satisfaction subscale scores progressed towards their maximum level. Cook and Campbell (1979 p.52) call this phenomenon the 'ceiling effect'. They point out that it leads to there being little possibility of further improvement at post-test. As Metcalfe (1982) asked in her study "if job satisfaction is already quite high...is it reasonable to expect it to go higher?" (p.359).

Nonetheless, one could ask why was nurse satisfaction so high that the 'ceiling effect' occurred. It could be that the questionnaire was not sensitive enough or that staff on both wards artificially inflated their scores to please the researcher. A more worrying explanation could have been that their expectations about patient care on a long-stay ward were so low that they were very satisfied with the pre-test care they were giving. However these explanations are only tentative and non-significant findings of this kind will be discussed in more detail below.

When total staff satisfaction scores were subjected to the Wilcoxon test (table 12.9) a significant change in Ward X's scores between pre-test and post-test was noted. This supports the opinions of several British authors that nurse satisfaction would be an inevitable result of working with a nursing model (Green, 1985; Salvage and Kershaw, 1990).

Although the Mann-Whitney results were mixed (see figure 12.13) the staff on Ward X had a better score on the attitude towards nursing models questionnaire than their counterparts on Ward Y. This was supported by the findings from the Wilcoxon test (see table 12.10) which indicated that between pre-test and post-test the staff on Ward X significantly increased their score. This also coincides with the opinions expressed by respondents in part one of this study and the findings of American studies reviewed in chapter three (Hagmiere and Hunt, 1979; Jacobson, 1987).

The total NOSIE score on Ward X increased steadily over the research period. In contrast the total score on Ward Y decreased over the same period (fig 12.14). Nonetheless the results of the Mann-Whitney U test and the Wilcoxon test can best be described as mixed. These results would imply that, according to registered nurses who knew them, the patients' behaviour on Ward X did not significantly change. Perhaps the inveterate behaviour of long-stay psychiatric patients cannot easily be changed. When Guy and Moore (1982) applied NOSIE in an American long-stay psychiatric facility they found that "when dealing with chronic psychiatric inpatients...the maintenance of appropriate behaviour is the maximum progress that can be expected." (p.22). They also found that non significant results may have occurred not because the patients did not improve, but because they did not improve as much as anticipated. This was a possibility in the present study.

The substantial improvement in dependency levels among patients in Ward X has some support in the literature. At post-test the external assessors in the present study observed that Ward Y was very traditional while Ward X was more patient centred. Miller (1989b) found that patients were less dependent when nursed on wards where the care was patient centred rather than routinized. Further, Torres (1989) gave a good overview of models that have human needs as their central theme. She pointed out that most of them were concerned with increasing the patient's independence concerning these human needs. It is also noteworthy that the originators of the HNM state that it acts by encouraging patient independence (Minshull et al, 1986).

The prescribing patterns for medications were monitored on both wards over the research period. Results showed that there were more medications being prescribed on Ward X than on Ward Y. But when interpreting this dissimilarity the greater number of patients on Ward X must be considered. When both wards were compared statistically there was no across-ward variation in prescribing patterns for psychotrophic medications. This result has important implications for other findings. It can be stated with some degree of confidence that positive changes in the other dependent variables were not the result of changes in medication prescribing pattern over the research period.

Results discussed above and depicted in table 12.19 show that the patients on Ward X were improving psychologically and socially. However their medication pattern did not change over the research period. One could ask if the consultants had been aware of these results would they have reduced the patients' medication. However, because the data were not analysed until the field work was complete, the consultants were not made aware of these results. Therefore although the HNM was introduced and it appeared to be having some effect the application of the medical model of therapy had remained the same. This apparent eclecticism within the HNM will be discussed in greater detail below.

*Possible threats to the validity of the findings*

For most of the dependent variables on Ward X it was possible to reject the null hypotheses and accept the research hypotheses. These results suggest a positive relationship between the implementation of the HNM and quality of care as measured by the research instruments used. This would support the assertions of many authors who suggest that nursing models can influence the improvement in quality of patient care (Engstrom, 1984; Green, 1985; Herbert, 1986; Jackson, 1986; Storch, 1986; Fawcett, 1989).

The ability to infer that an independent variable caused the change in dependent variables is termed internal validity. Within a quasi-experimental design Cook and Campbell (1979) argue that it is not possible to make confident conclusions until all the threats to internal validity are plausibly eliminated (p.55). The following threats to internal validity have been identified by Polit and Hungler (1987): history, selection, maturation, testing and mortality.

*History* refers to those events external to the independent variable that occur concurrently with it and can affect the dependent variables. *Selection* refers to the biases resulting from pre-test differences between experimental and control groups. *Maturation* refers to processes occurring within subjects during the study as a result of time rather than as a result of the independent variable. *Testing* refers to the biases that may result from respondents becoming familiar with or sensitized to issues within the research instruments. *Mortality* refers to the attrition of subjects from either the experimental or control group.

Cook and Campbell (1979) identify other threats to internal validity. For instance the collusion among subjects in an experimental group to improve artificially their results. This may be a result of their perception that the independent variable should have positive results. Conversely, subjects in a control group may become apathetic and frustrated with their perceived secondary role. Cook and Campbell call this *Resentful Demoralization*. Paradoxically, resentment in a control group may encourage imitation or a false inflation of scores. Cook and Campbell refer to these threats as *Imitation* and *Compensatory Rivalry* respectively. Within the study attempts were made to control the threats to internal validity.

In the present study the effects of History, Testing, Mortality, Selection and a desire to please the researcher were controlled by the presence of a control ward and by both wards having statistically similar pre-test scores. Selection was an important extraneous variable in the present study. But results from research into the effect of baseline differences between experimental groups question this importance. Lana found that "pre-test sensitization is probably less of a threat than was previously feared." (Cited in Cook and Campbell, 1979; p42).

There were other extraneous variables that must be considered. For instance, it was possible that patients and staff on Ward X deliberately skewed their responses in a positive direction. The motive may have been one of pride in their involvement in the change. Jones (1987) suspected staff of doing this in her study into the social atmosphere on acute hospital wards in Manchester. It was also possible that 'resentful demoralization' by patients and staff on Ward Y led to them having a poorer score. This could have contributed to the significant Mann-Whitney results on Ward X. But in order for these two alternative explanations to be valid there would have had to be collusion among most of the patients and staff on Ward X to increase their score and among those on Ward Y to decrease theirs. This scenario was unlikely and there was no evidence to suggest that it occurred.

In her research Miller (1989b) suggested that the personality, education and experience of the ward manager may affect the introduction of a care innovation. The ward sister on ward X who was acting as internal change agent was undertaking a psychology degree and had a positive commitment to the study. This motivation on her part could have encouraged an enthusiastic 'mind set' towards the HNM and towards staff and patient cohesiveness on the ward. To control for her 'mortality' an extra post-test (post-test1) was introduced once she left the ward. Results show that dependent variable scores continued to increase after her withdrawal from the study. This could, however, have been a result of the momentum for change she generated.

It was possible that 'maturation' may have had an effect on the results with patients and staff on Ward X growing wiser, more experienced and more perceptive between pre-test and post-test. It was also possible that the patients and staff on Ward X could have had their expectations increased by the preparations involved in introducing the HNM. This may have had the effect of inflating the scores on the dependent variables simply because they believed that this should occur. Discussing his experiment Barker (1988) refers to this phenomenon as the 'plausibility' factor. The reverse may have been true of staff and patients on ward Y. They could have expected to do less well than Ward X and so a self fulfilling prophecy came true. However on no occasion did the researcher lead staff or patients on either ward to believe that the use of the HNM would lead to better results.

There are other questions that merit consideration: could it be that using the HNM led to a renewed interest in the nursing process and it was the nursing process that made the difference to the dependent variables? Could it also be that the use of the action research approach made the difference? If so is it possible that any nursing model introduced in this way would have similar effects? Other than trying to control for these variables in a replicative study there is no way of answering these questions.

In summary, extraneous variables were controlled as far as was possible. In addition it was decided to reduce the possibility of making a type I error by lowering the alpha level from .05 to .02 for the Wilcoxon test.

Polit and Hungler (1987) support the non-equivalent control group approach as one of the most robust quasi-experimental designs available. However they stress that it is seldom possible to rule out all possible competing explanations for significant results. Therefore, although most of the threats to internal validity are implausible they cannot all be totally repudiated as competing reasons for the results. This reduces, but does not eliminate, the possibility that the improvements to the dependent variables on Ward X were related to the use of the HNM.

*Alternative explanations for the non significant findings*

For some of the findings from Ward X there was not enough evidence to reject the null hypothesis and so a non significant result was achieved. These include the Mann-Whitney results for NOSIE and nurse satisfaction. Although non-significant results are difficult to interpret it is important to try to identify possible explanations for them. The following explanations merit consideration.

There may genuinely not have been an improvement in a particular dependent variable on Ward X. This could be because the theoretical basis for the study (that the use of nursing models improves quality of care) was faulty. However descriptive results indicate that apart from medication patterns all the dependent variables showed some improvement on Ward X over the research period. Perhaps therefore improvement occurred but it was not large enough to be statistically significant at the predetermined alpha level.

It is also possible that a longer period may have been required for a statistically significant improvement in Ward X's score to occur or that the non-parametric test

212

used was not robust enough to detect the improvement. Also, a type II error may have been committed and the null hypothesis was not rejected when it should have been. This may have been the result of insufficient power where a larger sample would have been required to show a statistically significant improvement in Ward X's score. Polit and Hungler (1987) state that "The majority of nursing research studies in which the null hypothesis is not rejected are the consequences of insufficient power." (p.485).

Paradoxically, another explanation for a non-significant result on Ward X may have been due to an increase in the scores on Ward Y. This may have been due to 'imitation' or 'compensatory rivalry' (Cook and Campbell, 1979). This would have made it more difficult to get a statistically significant result on Ward X when scores were compared by the Mann-Whitney U test. Moreover, since the staff on Ward Y knew the researcher was interested in nursing models they may have been trying to please him by inflating their score. However this explanation could equally be applied to staff on Ward X. Nevertheless it was possible that perceptions about nursing models really did improve among staff on Ward Y due to the study stimulating a renewed interest in such frameworks.

On Ward X out of the eleven dependent variables examined there was a non-significant Wilcoxon result for five of them for the period post-test1 to post-test2. This occurred with the staff WAS, patient monitor, nurse satisfaction questionnaire, attitudes towards nursing models and the NOSIE. Although these findings did not affect the acceptance of the null hypothesis (H[1]b) they do need examination.

Most of the possible explanations for non-significant findings have been discussed above but in specifically dealing with this aberration the following reasons seem warranted. There may have been a lowering of morale in the post-test1 to post-test2 period. This could have been due to the 'loss' of the internal change agent or the movement of staff for 'cover' purposes during the January 1990 influenza epidemic. This could have caused a slowing down (rather than a reversal) in the rate of score improvement and contributed to some of the non-significant findings on Ward X. The ceiling effect may also have had an influence on the post-test1 to post-test2 scores (see p.208). A more serious reason for this result could have been the possibility that staff on Ward X were slowly tiring of nursing models in general and the HNM in particular. These are tentative suggestions and, without further research, must be accepted as such.

*The generalizability of the findings.*

External validity refers to the ability to generalize a study's findings to other settings or samples. This ability forms an important part of the interpretation of findings. Polit and Hungler (1987) describe the following threats to external validity: the Hawthorne effect, the novelty effect, the experimenter effect and the measurement effect.

Within this study control of the Hawthorne effect was attempted in two main ways. Prior to collecting pre-test data two weeks were spent on both wards letting patients and staff get used to the researcher's presence. Further, as much as possible, throughout the research period an equal amount of time was spent on Ward X and Ward Y. The 'novelty effect' may appear to be a considerable threat but staff on both wards had used nursing models before and as Polit and Hungler (1987) point out the novelty effect wears off when the new treatment becomes more familiar.

There was always the possibility that, however subconscious, the 'experimenter effect' affected the data collection procedure. One attempt to control this effect was to get persons other than the researcher to complete the research instruments. This was done with the following instruments: the nurse satisfaction questionnaire; the attitudes towards models questionnaire; the staff 'real' and 'ideal' ward atmosphere scale (WAS); the nurses' observation scale for inpatient evaluation (NOSIE); the patient dependency scale; and the armitage assessment instrument (AAI). The 'measurement effect' is difficult to control and its influence can only really be determined by replication.

Striving to assure internal validity by exerting a high degree of control over extraneous variables may make the research situation so distinctive that external validity is impossible. Although the threats to external validity were controlled as far as was possible in this study, gaining internal validity was seen as more important. Therefore a decision was made that internal validity would not be sacrificed in an attempt to obtain external validity. Campbell and Stanley (1973) recommend such a decision.

Macleod-Clarke and Hockey (1979) question whether the results from action research can be generalized at all. It can be recalled from the literature review that the use of a nursing model is unique to each ward and hospital. Moreover, the use of a nursing model can only be as effective as the institutional support it receives, so the ability to generalize the findings will always be limited to the degree of comparability between the research setting and the adopting ward or hospital. If the HNM is applied in a similar way in a similar setting there are indications that positive changes in the specified dependent variables may occur.

*Therapeutic eclecticism within the HNM*

While primarily using the HNM to structure their care nurses also appeared to be using (almost subconsciously) aspects of non-nursing models. For example nurses used aspects of: the supportive psychotherapeutic model when in one to one interaction with some patients, the behavioural model through positive reinforcement for good behaviour, the social model through groupwork and community visits and the medical model through the distribution of medications and the reporting of side effects. Barber (1986) believed such a repertoire was important. He suggested that without an ability to establish therapeutic relations nursing models will fail to thrive and remain at the level of filling in the kardex in a new way.

According to the literature (see p.13) eclecticism is a normal, even preferable, occurrence among psychiatric nurses. Walsh (1991) suggests that nursing models on their own cannot provide a sufficient knowledge base for patient care. He continues by stating that nursing models:

> ...facilitate the bringing together of knowledge from a wide range of other disciplines to supplement the core nursing knowledge required for quality nursing care." (p.5).

It would appear that the ability to be therapeutically eclectic existed among staff on both research wards prior to the commencement of the study. However when staff on Ward X began to use the HNM they naturally drew more on these skills to help the patient towards independence in the five levels of human need. This does not detract from the HNM. It acted as a broad nursing framework within which some nursing and non-nursing intervention strategies were employed. With the HNM these skills had the opportunity to emerge rather than remain dormant.

Although the HNM encouraged the emergence of other non-nursing models for intervention purposes it has been pointed out elsewhere that the medical influence did not change on either ward over the research period. Considering the fact that the medical staff only visited the research wards one day per week this tenacity to medical routines is surprising. However it could be argued that although medications continued to be prescribed and distributed they did not have the same importance for staff on Ward X. To them medications were seen as another therapeutic regime like supportive psychotherapy and not as an all consuming framework for patient care.

*Power redistribution*

Previous research suggested that the proper implementation of a nursing model requires a hierarchal redistribution of power (Keyzer, 1985). In the present study there appeared to be a shift of power from nurse management to ward staff. There was also a shift of power from ward staff to patients. The manifestation of this power

215

took the form of the confidence to make decisions. Nurses on Ward X were also more able to: become involved, to question, to redesign documentation, to propose and undertake new therapies, to justify their judgments to medical colleagues, to be different from other long-stay wards, to challenge the researcher and much more. Patient power took the form of their involvement in care planning, having new assertiveness and self awareness skills and having a choice in purchasing items such as clothes.

This redistribution of power is at odds with the traditional medical model approach to nursing care. It was to their credit that all the managers and practising nurses in the present study supported it. A possible reason for this support may lie in the make up of the HNM itself. Compared to the more extreme American nursing models, the HNM does not call for a radical change in thinking among patients and staff (perhaps this was a reason for its selection in the first place). This perception of it being a small step away from the 'status quo' may have made it more acceptable to nurse managers and thus made them more willing to redistribute power. Regardless of the possible reasons for the 'power shift', the nurse and patient on Ward X held more power at post-test than at pre-test. It is possible that this power took the form of what Pearson (1985) called 'delegated power'. Patients and ward nurses possessed it because managers allowed them to have it.

But it is questionable whether the medical staff redistributed any of their power. They gave their endorsement to the change; they did not interfere with it and made no attempt to sabotage it. Yet, although welcome, they made no attempt to actively be part of the change. Therefore it could be suggested that the medical staff allowed the nursing staff to introduce an innovation but throughout its introduction the medical input remained the same.

*Reflection on the action research approach*

As an approach to data collection action research has been discussed in detail in chapter twelve. The decision to use it was a worthwhile one. It became obvious that change would not have been possible without the involvement of patients and staff; a text book application of a quasi-experimental design would not have worked.

It is possible that for some staff the action research approach was threatening. It leads to questioning of current comfortable practices. However in the present study the change to a democratic form of decision making appeared to be relatively painless for the participants. It is highly likely that this was due to the diligence by which the internal change agents adopted this role. Although a collaborative study the staff or patients were not involved in the analysis of data. They agreed that the data belonged, at least temporarily, to the researcher. Failure to resolve the issue of ownership of data could have implications for collaborative research (Meyer, 1992).

In the present study it was rewarding to see the patients and staff wanting and accepting ownership of the change. This ensured a possessiveness and allegiance to the change that would not have occurred through imposition. Perhaps the key to the action research approach was education, collaboration and open discussion. These elements are rarely seen in the power-coercive change strategy. The researcher believes that the use of the action research approach led to an increase in research mindedness among the staff. It also enriched the personal and professional development of all those involved.

**Limitations**

Most research studies in nursing are liable to certain limitations because their field of interest is human activity which by definition is an unpredictable area of investigation. The present study was no exception and the relevant limitations as perceived by the researcher are outlined below. There were also certain delimitations placed on the study prior to entering the research area. These included restricting the study to:

1. long stay psychiatric care;

2. a Northern Ireland context;

3. one large psychiatric hospital;

4. two long stay psychiatric wards;

5. nursing staff and patients only;

6. those respondents who were willing and able to take part;

7. those responses that participants were aware of and were willing to express.

*Instrumentation*

Lancaster and Lancaster (1981) and Walsh (1990) pointed out that there were no suitable tools available to evaluate the effectiveness of nursing models. In retrospect most of those chosen were limited by the absence of open ended questions which

217

could have led to the collection of richer data. Further, five of the instruments were of the self report variety. In his research Barker (1988) explains the problems with this type of instrument but concludes that self report is an important way of exploring experiences.

*Sample*

The small size of the patient and staff groups suggest that care must be taken in drawing conclusions from the findings. The size of the groups was influenced partly by the limited number of patients and staff on the research wards and partly by the exclusion and withdrawal of a few respondents from the study. Paradoxically, given the small sample size, the presence of significant post-test findings suggests very real differences between the groups in dependent variable scores.

Random selection of patients to control and experimental groups was not possible and any attempt to do so could be said to be practically and ethically untenable. Even though Ward X and Ward Y were matched for a range of variables, the noncomparability for the variable gender may have affected the results. Hanley et al (1981) and Barker (1988) reported sex differences in patient responses to dementia and depression respectively. However there is no discussion in the literature regarding the relationship between nursing models and gender. Therefore, without further research, there is no way of knowing if such an effect occurred and if so what influence it had on the findings.

It could be argued that the professional competencies of nurses are critical to model efficacy. Although the researcher was aware of the level of competency staff had about nursing models, more general actual or potential nurse competencies were not appraised at pre-test. Such an appraisal would have been difficult to undertake. Therefore there is no way of knowing if level of competency had an effect on the use of the HNM.

*Implementing the HNM*

Previous research into British psychiatric nursing pointed out that six months was too short a time scale to implement a care innovation (Cadbury, 1980; Barker, 1988; Armitage, 1990). For this reason approximately nine months was chosen as the time span for the present study. Although significant changes in dependent variables were noted within this period it was barely adequate when preparation for change, education for change, introduction of the change and evaluation of the change were considered. This could have been an influencing factor for some of the non significant findings.

218

*Data collection*

Even though most patient care data were collected by the researcher a very real attempt was made to eliminate bias in the mode of questioning and in the completion of the instruments. However it is not known if the researcher subconsciously inflicted his own impression on the way a question should be answered by intonations of voice. External assessors were used for the AAI as blind raters. It was recognized that they could also have been used in the application of ward monitor and patient monitor. Pressure on their time militated against this strategy. However even the employment of a second investigator to control for variation in the assessment of these tools would have strengthened the reliability of the results. Furthermore, inter-rater reliability for the external assessors was not estimated. Failure to do any of these could be considered a methodological flaw.

Because the NOSIE and the patient dependency scales were completed by the patients' key nurses it was possible that their scores may be influenced by the perceptions the nurses have of particular patients. If the opinion of Miller (1989b) is accepted this may be particularly true. She states that nurses working on traditional wards tend to overestimate patient dependency levels while nurses working on more individualized wards tend to underestimate the patient's dependency (p.379). The potential for subjectivity of this kind must be recognized when drawing conclusions from these results.

*Research approach*

This study combines quasi-experimental and action research approaches. The potential limitations of such a combination have already been discussed in chapter eleven. Research theorists argue that investigators should use a mix of approaches. The choice should be made according to what is best suited to the research needs and not according to the method's traditional affiliations. Both qualitative and quantitative research deserve credit as rigorous scientific methodologies. Nonetheless a pure ethnographic approach with the researcher joining groups of nurses and monitoring changes as they happened would perhaps have resulted in stronger data.

*Analysis of data*

Pre-test equivalency between the two wards regarding age, length of stay and most of the dependent variables was shown statistically. However lack of equivalency at pre-test for patient dependency limits the validity of its findings.

Results from Ward X indicate that the HNM may have had a significant effect (in a positive direction) on the dependent variables. However there is no indication of the size of the effect. Although the graphical presentation of data does show a larger effect on Ward X, a calculation of confidence intervals could have supplied more precise information concerning size of effect.

Sometimes when carrying out research there is a strong temptation to wander from the area under investigation and conduct tangential data analysis exercises. Such diversions can be seductive to a researcher. Time permitting, it would have been interesting to compare the responses of day and night staff or the patients' and staffs' perception of the ward atmosphere. It would also have been interesting to examine if trained staffs' use of the HNM create a new subservient role for untrained staff. Furthermore, in the data presentation chapter, total scores rather than subscale scores were compared using inferential statistics and the semi-interquartile range was not reported. Reporting any of these extra analyses would have increased the length of the thesis substantially, while adding little to the findings.

## Conclusions

Taking into account the threats to internal validity and the limitations outlined above the following conclusions are identified. These are stated regarding the study's hypotheses. However serendipitous conclusions not directly related to the hypotheses will also be included.

### Conclusions from the research hypotheses

Results suggest that after the introduction of the HNM on a long-stay psychiatric ward positive changes in specific indicators of Structure, Processes and Outcomes of care occurred. Therefore when compared to Ward Y the results from Ward X suggest that:

*Structure*

1. the significant improvement in ward structure as measured by ward monitor, WAS and the AAI was related to the introduction of the HNM;

*Process*

2. the significant improvement in care processes as measured by patient monitor and care plan goals was related to the introduction of the HNM;

*Outcome*

3.  the significant improvement in care outcomes as measured by patient satisfaction questionnaire, attitudes towards models questionnaire and patient dependency scale was related to the introduction of the HNM;

4.  Improvement in psychosocial aspects of patient care, as measured by constituents within the research instruments, was related to the introduction of the HNM;

5.  results suggest that when compared with a control ward the improvement in two of the outcome measures (nurse satisfaction and NOSIE) was not large enough to be significant;

6.  there was no significant difference between wards in the prescribing of psycho-trophic medication over the research period.

These conclusions contribute to contemporary theoretical thinking on the positive relationship between nursing models and quality of care.

*Conclusions from serendipitous findings*

1.  an    action research approach is a powerful method for introducing a nursing model into clinical practice and a combination of research methods can lead to the enrichment of a study;

2.  the need for management    support, medical staff endorsement and in-service education is crucial for the successful introduction of a nursing model;

3.  the need for a 'downward' redistribution of power (albeit delegated power) is necessary for the proper implementation of nursing models;

4.  the contribution of change theory and planned change to the introduction of a nursing model are significant;

5.  internal change agents with support from an external change agent and regular staff meetings strengthen the change strategy and contribute to a model's introduction;

6.  the implementation of a nursing model is made easier if the model is adapted to suit the patient care setting;

7. the change to model based practice should be a partnership between patients, practitioners, managers and educators;

8. although the staff used the HNM to assess, plan, implement and evaluate patient care, some eclectic features of non-nursing models were also used as intervention strategies.

## Implications

The findings of this study may be of value to the nursing community. However, by their very nature, implications are often speculative and so the following are expressed in tentative terms.

### Implications for practising psychiatric nurses

The findings suggest the existence of a positive relationship between using the HNM and specific indicators of care quality. Furthermore the introduction of the HNM appears to positively affect those specified psychosocial aspects of patient care. Practising nurses should be aware of these findings and use them to improve patient care and the status of long-stay psychiatric wards. Therefore nurses working within long-stay psychiatric wards should use a suitable nursing model to assess, plan, implement and evaluate the care of their patients.

Findings indicate that the HNM model can act as an general framework of care within which other non-nursing models can be used for intervention purposes. Therefore the nurse is not rejecting interventions that may be useful simply because they do not originate from nursing. Rather, the practising nurse can select whatever therapeutic tools she believes she requires to achieve the patient centred goals leading to independence in human needs. This may lead nurses to have their own theoretical underpinning but also be able to practice in a collaborative way with other health professionals.

Unlike psychiatrists nurses do not have a repertoire of physical treatments which they can use with patients. Nurses must use themselves as therapeutic agents. However many do not do this (Altschul, 1981). Any innovation that appears to enable psychiatric nurses to improve the care they give to patients and increase their therapeutic status should be grasped. Results of the present study demonstrate that, when properly implemented, a nursing model has the ability to achieve these goals. If replications of this study support the present findings this may give practising nurses more power to influence patient care.

However this empowerment of staff has further implications. Practising nurses and patients may not be ready or willing to accept power. Some may be afraid of the extra responsibility and accountability that such power will bring. Furthermore nurses may not be willing to give the patients more power as this could undermine the practitioners' authority (see p.12). These are important professional issues that may be solved by education and support. However the wishes of those patients and nurses who do not want more power should be respected.

*Implications for nurse educators*

Hollingworth (1985) maintained that new conduct for nurses often requires new knowledge, new skills, new attitudes and a new value orientation. A change towards using nursing models for psychiatric patient care is unlikely to take place in the absence of educational support. No matter how impressed ward staff may be with a particular nursing model if they do not receive proper education for its implementation their knowledge base will be too unsteady to sustain such an innovation.

Nurses also require 'informed role models' to instigate and encourage model based practice. Therefore nurse teachers should not merely concentrate on educating staff in class rooms but also have a ward based educational input with staff nurses, enrolled nurses and nursing auxiliaries. In this role teachers could act as joint change agents with ward managers. However, it should not be taken for granted that all nurse teachers have the necessary skills to adopt such a role. In this regard the UKCC should be prepared to introduce programmes to 'teach the teachers'.

It would be educationally restrictive for nurse teachers to 'sell' a model as the panacea to all nursing's ills. Rather they must point out that no one model answers all nursing questions. Thus although the HNM is broad enough for widespread acceptance and application in long-stay psychiatric nursing it should be introduced with other models to students and practitioners alike. It must not also be seen as a replacement for all medically, psychologically or socially orientated interventions. Nurse educators must respect eclecticism among practising nurses.

*Implications for managers*

To introduce a nursing model ward staff require management support. Provided that patient safety has priority, nurses must be allowed time and latitude to take chances with new ideas. If such allowances do not take place ward staff may be afraid to abandon safe routines in case they find that they cannot cope with the new model or in case they make some error that might get them into legal difficulties. If models are applied rigidly rather than as flexible instruments of care the nurse will be constrained within a legalistic straitjacket.

The Griffith's management structure (1984) has removed much of patient care from the control and management of nurses. It is uncertain whether these non-nurse managers are committed to the introduction of nursing models to practice. Their commitment may be influenced by the potential these frameworks have for the quality of care. The findings from this study indicate that the introduction of nursing models should have management priority.

*Implications for nurse theorists*

It was not until 1980 that models began to be produced in the United Kingdom. There are now twelve of these and it appears theorists here will mimic their American colleagues and produce more. A better theoretical strategy would be to introduce a moratorium (perhaps temporary) on model production and concentrate on the testing and evaluation of the existing models in practice. For example, the further systematic use of the HNM could help in the formulation of propositions which in turn could lead to testable hypotheses. In this way clinically useful micro theories could emanate from nursing models.

To conclude this section on implications it can be said that when implemented properly a nursing model can have a positive effect on the quality of the specific structures, processes and outcomes of psychiatric care. Therefore all nurses, whether in practice, education or management must work with patients and other professional colleagues to ensure that these models are selected, tested and used for the benefit of all concerned.

## Recommendations

Recommendations will be categorized into 'programmatic recommendations' that relate to the topic under study and 'further study recommendations' related to the limits of the present study and to new directions for research in the field.

Based upon the results of part two of the study, the following recommendations are suggested:

*Programmatic recommendations*

1.  The implementation of educational programmes within PREP that will help practising nurses understand and use nursing models;

2. Nursing models should be supported by nurse clinicians, managers and educators;

3. Within the health service internal change agents should be given an officially recognized role.

*Further research recommendations*

This area of study is far from being saturated on either side of the Atlantic. Therefore it is recommended that:

1. The study should be replicated on a variety of wards in different geographical areas with larger samples of patients and staff. This would provide a population large enough for more exacting analysis;

2. The relationship between gender and nursing models should be explored;

3. More reliable and valid quality assurance tools for psychiatric nursing should be developed. A mixture of open and closed ended questions should be included;

4. The instruments used require further psychometric testing and there should be more valid and reliable instruments specifically available to evaluate the use of nursing models;

5. A longitudinal study with a longer time frame should be used to evaluate change to model based practice; at least one year;

6. External assessors blind to the independent variable and appraised for inter-rater reliability should be used to collect the data;

7. Future research should attempt to control the nursing competencies or make comparisons between wards where the staff competencies are high and wards where the staff are less competent;

8. Research should be undertaken to discover how eclectic are psychiatric nurses and do they use eclecticism consciously or subconsciously;

9. The action research approach should be used as a way of linking practice with research and theory and for the implementation of innovations. The practising nurse should be actively involved in these endeavours;

10.   A range of qualitative research methods should be used for a more in-depth exploration of the change to a nursing model. Grounded theory, repertory grid technique and Flanagan's critical incident technique may uncover rich data relating to how nursing models are implemented.

## Coda

It may be recalled (see p.172) that towards the completion of the data collection process there was a rumour on the research wards that they were going to close. This did happen on 24th June 1991 when both wards were converted into an administration block. Most of the patients were transferred to other wards.

The closure of Apple villa raises ethical questions that are of concern to the researcher. Is it possible that some of the patients connected the study with the subsequent closure of their 'home'? Could some of the staff have had similar thoughts? Furthermore the HNM as introduced on Ward X stressed patient involvement in decision making. However the patients appeared to have had no part in their resettlement decision.

Since the completion of the study three staff have completed their general training and were returning, one has commenced a degree course and two have became community psychiatric nurses. This raises other questions: If Ward X had not closed would they have remained in the hospital? Did their involvement in the study stimulate a desire for further knowledge and professional advancement? Would this career progression have taken place if they had not been involved in the study? Unfortunately there are no answers to these questions. However, perhaps the research gave them an insight into their worth and helped whet their appetite for further study.

Generally the results of this study were encouraging. It is hoped that they will lead to a greater understanding about the selection and implementation of nursing models. It is also hoped that the study will contribute to the growing body of knowledge on nursing models in mental health and in the link between nursing models and quality of care.

# Bibliography

Abdellah, F.G. Beland, I.L. Martin, A. Matheney, R.V. (1960). *Patient centred approaches to nursing*. New York, Macmillan.

Adam, E.T. (1975). A conceptual model for nursing. *The Canadian Nurse*, 71(14) :40-43.

Adam, E.T. (1980). *To be a nurse*. New York, W.B. Saunders.

Adam, E.T. (1983). Frontiers of nursing in the 21st century: development of models and theories on the concept of nursing. *Journal of Advanced Nursing*, 8(1) :41-45.

Adam, E.T. (1985). Towards more clarity in terminology: frameworks, theories and models. *Journal of Nurse Education*, 24(4) :151-155.

Adelson, P.Y. (1980). The back ward dilemma. *American Journal of Nursing*, 80 :423-425.

Aggleton, P. Chalmers, H. (1986). *Nursing models and the nursing process*. Basingstoke, MacMillan Ed.

Aggleton, P.J. Chalmers, H.A. (1987). Nursing research, nursing theory and the nursing process. *Journal of Advanced Nursing*, 12(5) :573-581.

Aggelton, P. Chalmers, C. (1990). Nursing models: model future. *Nursing Times*, 86(3) :41-43.

Alexandrer, M. Orton,H. (1988). Research in action. *Nursing Times*, 84(8) :38-41.

Ali, L (1990). Models in accident and emergency. *Nursing Standard*, 5(4) :21-24.

Allen,M.N.Hayes,P.(1989).Models of nursing: implications for research in nursing. In Akinsanya, J. (ed). *Recent Advances in Nursing*, 24 :77-92.

Altschul,A.T. (1962). Trends in psychiatric nursing. In Freeman, H. Farndale, J. eds. *Trends in mental health services*. London, Pergamon Press.

Altschul, A.T. (1972). *Patient-nurse interaction. A study of interaction patterns in acute psychiatric wards*. Edinburgh, Churchill Livingstone.

Altschul, A.T. Simpson, R. (1977). *Psychiatric nursing*. London, Bailliere Tindall.

Altschul, A. T. (1978). A systems approach to the nursing process. *Journal of Advanced Nursing*, 3 :333-340.

Altschul, A.T. (1980). The care of the mentally disordered: three Approaches. *Nursing Times*, 76(11) :452-454.

Altschul, A.T. (1981). Issues in psychiatric nursing. In Hockey, L. (ed) *Current issues in nursing*. Edinburgh, Churchill Livingstone.

Altschul, A.T. (1983). The consumer's voice: nursing implications. *Journal of Advanced Nursing*, 8 :175-183.

Altschul, A.T. (1985). Introduction. In, Barker, P.J. & Fraser, D. *The nurse as a therapist: a behavioural model*. London, Croom Helm.

Anderson, P. (1986). The Delphi technique in practice. *Australian Journal of Advanced Nursing*, 3(2) :22-32.

Armitage, P. (1990).*An evaluation of primary nursing and the role of the nurse preceptor in changing long-term mental health care*. University of Wales, Unpublished Ph.D. thesis.

Armitage, P. Morrison, P. (1991). Changing behaviour. *Nursing Times*, 87(9) :33-35.

Auld, M.B. (1968). Team nursing in a maternity hospital. *Midwife & Health Visitor*, 4(15) :242-245.

Ayllon, T. Michael, J. (1959). The psychiatric nurse as a behavioural engineer. *Journal of the Experimental Analysis of Behaviour*, 2 :323-324.

Bagehot, W. (1873). In The Oxford dictionary of quotations, 3rd edition. London, Guild Publishing.

Baker, A.A. ed (1976). *Comprehensive psychiatric care*. Oxford, Blackwell Scientific Publications.

Ball, J.A. Goldstone, L.A. Collier, M.M. (1984). *Criteria for care: the manual of the North West Nurse Staffing Levels Project*. Newcastle-upon-Tyne, Newcastle-Upon -Tyne Products Ltd.

Baly, M.E. (1979). *Nursing and social change*. 2nd ed. London, Heinemann.

Bandura, A. (1969). *Principles of behaviour modification*. London, Holt Rinehart & Winston.

Barber, P (1986). The psychiatric nurse's failure therapeutically to nurture. *Nursing Practice*, 1(3) :138-141.

Barber, P. ed. (1990). *Mental handicap*. Choosing a model series. London, Edward Arnold.

Barker, P.J. (1982). *Behaviour therapy nursing*. London, Croom Helm.

Barker, P.J. Fraser, D. Eds. (1985). *The nurse as a therapist: a behavioural model*. London, Croom Helm.

Barker, P.J. (1988). *An evaluation of specific nursing interventions in the management of patients suffering from manic depressive psychosis*. Dundee College of Technology. Unpublished Ph.D thesis.

Barker, P.J. (1990). The conceptual basis of mental health nursing. *Nurse Education Today*, 10 :339-348.

Barker, P.J. (1991). Finding common ground. *Nursing Times*, 87(2) :37-38.

Baron, R. Bryne, D. (1984). *Social psychology: understanding human interaction.* Boston, Allyn & Bacon Inc.

Barton, R. (1959). *Institutional neurosis.* Bristol, John Wright & Sons.

Beard, M.T. Enelow, C.T. Owens, J.G. (1978). Activity therapy as a reconstructive plan on the social competence of chronic hospitalised patients. *Journal of Psychiatric Nursing and Mental Health Services,* 16(12) :33-41.

Beck, A.T. (1976). *Cognitive therapy: the emotional disorders.* New York, University Press.

Beck, C.T. (1985). Theoretical frameworks cited in Nursing Research from January 1974-June 1985. *Nurse Educator*, 10(6) :36-38.

Beckstrand, J. (1980). A critique of several conceptions of practice theory in nursing. *Research in Nursing and Health,* 3(2) :69-80.

Bendall, E. (1975). *So you passed, nurse.* London. Royal College of Nursing.

Bennis, W.G. Benne, K.D. Chin, R. Corey, K.E. (1976). *The planning of change.* 3rd ed. New York, Holt, Rinhart and Winston.

Bentley, J. Boojawon, D. (1990). Measuring quality in a psychiatric hospital. *Nursing Times*, 86(42) :46-48.

Bevvino, C.A. Burns, B. Lewis, M.H. Allen, J.K. (1984). Planned change: an innovative nursing rehabilitation model. *Perspectives in Psychiatric Care*, XXll(4) :149-158.

Biley, F. (1991). The divide between theory and practice. *Nursing,* 4(29) :30-33.

Bird, J. Marks, I.M. Lindley, P. (1979). Nurse therapists in psychiatry: some developments, controversies and implications. *British Journal of Psychiatry,* 135 :321-329.

Bishop, S.M. (1986). History and philosophy of science. In, Marriner, A. ed. *Nursing theorists and their Work.* St Louis, C.V. Mosby.

Bloch, D. (1975). Evaluation of nursing care in terms of process and outcome. Issues in research and quality assurance. *Nursing Research,* 24(4) :256-263.

Blumer, H. (1969). *Symbolic interactionism: perspective and method.* New Jersey, Prentice Hall, Englewood Cliffs.

Bogdanovic, A. (1989). Non-verbal communication. *Nursing Times*, 85(1) :27-28.

Bohny, B. (1980). Theory development for a nursing science. *Nursing Forum,* 19(1) :50-67.

Bokholdt, M.G. Kanters, H.W. (1978). Team nursing in a general hospital - theory, results and limitations. *Journal of Occupational Psychology*, 51 :315-325.

Bond, S. Bond, J. (1982). A Delphi survey of clinical nursing research priorities. *Journal of Advanced Nursing*, 7(6) :565-576.

Boore, J.R.P. (1978). *A prescription for recovery.* London, Royal College of Nursing.

Botha, M.E. (1989). Theory development in perspective: the role of conceptual frameworks and models in theory development. *Journal of Advanced Nursing*, 14 :49-55.

Bouras, N. Trauer, T. Watson, (1982). Ward environment and disturbed behaviour. *Psychological Medicine,* 12(2) :309-319.

Bowers, L. (1989). The significance of primary nursing. *Journal of Advanced Nursing*, 14 :13-19.

Bowman, G.S. Thompson, D.R. Sutton, T.W. (1983). Nurses' attitudes towards the nursing process. *Journal of Advanced Nursing*, 8 :125-129.

Bramwell, L. Hykawy, E. (1974). The Delphi technique: a possible tool for predicting future events in nurse education. *Nursing Papers* (Can), 6(1) :23-32.

Brewster, M. Cook, M. Woodward, S. (1991). *Standard care plan system: critical but stable*. Oxford, Paper presented at the Quality Assurance Network Conference.

Bronowski, J. (1980). The ascent of man. London, BBC.

Brooker, C.G. (1986). Some problems associated with the measurement of community psychiatric nurse intervention. *Journal of Advanced Nursing*, 9 :165-174.

Brooking, J.I. (1984). *Current provision for advanced psychiatric nursing education*. Sheffield, Paper presented at the Association of Integrated and Degree Courses in Nursing's Annual Conference.

Brooking, J. ed (1986). *Psychiatric nursing research*. Chichester, John Wiley & Sons.

Brooking. J. (1986). *Patient and family participation in nursing care: the development of a nursing process measuring scale*. College, London, Unpublished Ph.D Thesis.

Brymer, A. Cramer, D. (1990). *Quantitative data analysis for social scientists*. London, Routledge.

Burgess, A.C. Lazare, A. (1973). *Psychiatric nursing in the hospital and the community*. New Jersey, Prentice Hall, Englewood Cliffs :108-122.

Burnard, P. (1990). Thoughts about theories. *Nursing Standard*, 4(21) :47.

Butler, R.J. Rosenthal, G. (1985). *Behaviour and rehabilitation*. 2nd ed. Bristol, John Wright & Sons.

Butterworth, T. (1991). Generating research in mental health nursing. *International Journal of Nursing Studies,* 28(3) :237-246.

Cadbury, S.J. (1980). *Assessment and change of the atmosphere on a psychiatric admission ward*. Dept of Psychiatry, University of Leeds, Unpublished M.Sc.

Campbell, D.T. Stanley, J.C. (1973). *Experimental and quasi-experimental designs for research*. Chicago, Rand McNally & Co.

Campbell, J.P. Dunnette, M.D. Lawler, E.E. Weick, K.E. (1974). Theories of motivation. In Dubin, R. (ed). *Human relations in administration* (4th ed). New Jersey, Prentice Hall.

Caplan, G. (1964). *Principles of preventive psychiatry*. New York, Basic Books Inc.

Carson, J. Shaw, L. Wills, W. (1989). Which patients first: a study from the closure of a large psychiatric hospital. *Health Trends,* 21 :117-120.

Cash. K. (1990). Nursing models and the idea of nursing. *International Journal of Nursing Studies,* 27(3) :249-256.

Castledine, G. (1986). A Stress adaptation model. In, Kershaw, B. Salvage, J, eds. *Models for nursing.* Chichester, John Wiley & Sons.

Chambers, H. (ed) (1988). *Cardiovascular and respiratory care. Choosing a model series.* London, Edward Arnold.

Chalmers, H. (1989). Theories and models of nursing and the nursing process. In Akinsanya J.A. (ed), *Theories and models of nursing.* Edinburgh, Churchill Livinstone.

Chapman, C.M. (1985). *Theory of nursing: practical application.* London, Harper and Row.

Chapman, P. (1990). A critical perspective. In Salvage, J. Kershaw, B. (eds) *Models for nursing 2.* London, Scutari Press.

Charlton, J.R.H. Patrick, D.L. Matthews, G. West, P.A. (1981). Spending priorities in Kent: a Delphi study. *Journal of Epidemiology and Community Health,* 35 :288-292.

Chavasse, J. (1978). From task assignment to patient allocation: a change evaluation. *Journal of Advanced Nursing,* 6 :137-145

Chavasse, J. (1987). A comparison of three models of nursing. *Nurse Education Today,* 7(4) :177-186.

Chein, I. Cook, S.W. Harding, J. (1948). The field of American research. *American Psychologist,* 3 :43-50.

Chin, R. Benne, K.D. (1976). General strategies for effecting change in human systems. In: Bennis, W.G. Benne, K.D. Chin, R. Corey, K.E. (1976). *The planning of change.* 3rd ed. New York, Holt, Rinhart and Winston.

Chinn, P. Jacobs, M. (1983, 1987). *Theory and nursing: a systematic approach.* St Louis, C.V. Mosby & Co.

Chong Choi, E. (1986) Evolution of nursing theory development. In, Marriner, A. ed, *Nursing theorists and their work.* St Louis, C.V. Mosby & Co.

Christie-Brown, J.R.W. Ebringer, L. Freedman, K.S. (1977). A survey of long-stay psychiatric population: implications for community services. *Psychological Medicine,* 7 :113-126.

Church, O.M. (1987). From custody to community in psychiatric nursing. *Nursing Research,* 36(1) :48-55.

Ciske, K.L. (1974). Primary nurse evaluation. *American J ournal of Nursing,* 74(8) :1436-1438.

Clare, A. (1976). *Psychiatry in dissent.* London, Tavistock Publishers.

Clark, J. (1982). Development of models and theories on the concept of nursing. *Journal of Advanced Nursing,* 7(1) :129-134.

231

Clark, J. (1986). A model for health visiting. In, Kershaw, B. Salvage, J. eds. *Models for nursing*. Chichester, John Wiley & Sons.

Clarke, M. (1986). Action and reflection: practice and theory in nursing. *Journal of Advanced Nursing*, 11 :3-11.

Clarke, J. (1991) Moral dilemmas in nursing research. *Nursing Practice* 4(4) :22-25.

Clinton, M. (1981). *Training psychiatric nurses. A sociological study of the problems of integrating theory and practice*. University of East Anglia, Unpublished Ph.D Thesis.

Cohen, J. Struening, E.L. (1965). Opinions about mental illness: hospital differences in attitudes for eight occupational groups. *Psychological Reports*, 17 :23-25.

Coleman, D.S. (1986). The issues as seen from the perspective of a director of nursing. In Wilkinson, G. Freeman, H. eds. *The provision of mental health services in Britain*. London, Gaskell.

Collins, V. (1975) *The primary nursing role as a model for evaluating quality of patient care, patient satisfaction, job satisfaction and cost effective in an acute care setting*. University of Utah, Unpublished PhD Thesis.

Collister, B. (1986). Psychiatric nursing and a developmental model. In Kershaw, B. Salvage, J. (eds). *Models for nursing*. Chichester, John Wiley & Sons.

Collister, B. (1988). *Psychiatric nursing: person to person*. London, Edward Arnold.

Cook, T.D. Campbell, D.T. (1979). *Quasi-experimentation: design and analysis issues for field setting*. Chicago, Rand McNally.

Cooper, F.E. (1988). *An evaluation of the nursing process used in the care of selected medical and surgical hospital patients*. University of Nottingham, Unpublished M.Phil Thesis.

Cope, D. Cox, S. (1980). Organisational development in a psychiatric hospital: creating desirable changes. *Journal of Advanced Nursing*, 5 :371-380.

Copeland, J.R.M. Wilson, K.C.M. (1989). Rating scales in old age psychiatry. In Thompson, C. (ed). *The instruments of psychiatric research*. Chichester, John Wiley & Sons.

Corey, L.J. Wallace, M.A. Harris, S.H. Casey, B. (1986). Psychiatric ward atmosphere. *Journal of Psychosocial Nursing,* 24(10) :10-16.

Corke, P. Cushion, B. Haddock, G. (1989). Resettlement of long-stay psychiatric patients. Occasional Paper. *Nursing Times*, 85(9) :44-46.

Cormack, D.F.S. (1976) *Psychiatric nursing observed*. London, Royal College of Nursing.

Cormack, D.F.S. (1981). *Psychiatric nursing described: an investigation of the role of the psychiatric nurse using Flanagan's Critical Incident technique*. Dundee College of Technology, Ph.D Thesis.

Cormack, D.F.S. (1983). *Psychiatric nursing described*. Edinburgh, Churchill Livingstone.

Corner, J. (1991). In search of more complete answers to research questions. Quantitative versus qualitative research methods: is there a way forward? *Journal of Advanced Nursing*, 16 :718-727.

Corrigan, J. Soni, S.D. (1977). Community psychiatric nursing: An appraisal of its impact on community psychiatry in Manchester. *Journal of Advanced Nursing*, 2 :347-354.

Corwin, R. (1961). The Professional employee: a study of conflict in nursing roles. *American Journal of Sociology*, 767 :604-615.

Cowan, S. (1986). In Webb,C. ed. *Womens health, midwifery and gynaecological nursing*. London, Hodder & Stoughton.

Craig, S.L. (1980). Theory development and its relevance for nursing. *Journal of Advanced Nursing*, 5 :349-355.

Crouch, S. (1990). The nursing process. *Nursing*, 4(12) :16-18.

Crow, J. (1977). *The nursing process*. London, Macmillan Journals Ltd.

Cummings, J. Cummings, E. (1962). *Ego and milieu: theory and practice of environmental therapy*. London, Tavistock.

Daeffler, R.J. (1975). Patient's perception of care under team and primary nursing. *Journal of Nursing Administration*, 5(3) :20.

Dalkey, N. Helmer, O. (1963). An experimental application of the Delphi method to the use of experts. *Management Science*, 9(3) :458-467.

Darcy, P.T. (1978). Psychiatric nursing today. 3. care conflicts. *Nursing Mirror*, 153(21) :26.

Darlington Memorial Hospital Inquiry (1976). *Report of the Committee of enquiry*. Newcastle, Northern Regional Health Authority.

Davis, C. (1976). Experience of dependency and control in work: the case of nurses. *Journal of Advanced Nursing*, 1(4) :273-282.

De la Cuesta (1979). *Nursing process: from theory to implementation*. University of London, Unpublished M.Sc Thesis.

Denn, R. (1975). Cited in Huey, F.L. *Psychiatric nursing 1946-1974: a report on the state of the art*. New York. The American Nursing Journal Co :11.

Denzin, N.K. (1970). *The research act: a theoretical introduction to sociological methods*. Chicago, Adine Publcations Co.

D.H.S.S. (1979). *Psychiatric hospitals in Northern Ireland. A study of physical facilities and estimates of future demands*. London, Her Majesty's Stationery Office.

D.H.S.S. (1979b). *Organisational and management problems of mental illness hospitals. Report of a working group*. Chairman: T.E. Nodder. London, Her Majesty's Stationery Office.

D.H.S.S. (1980). *Review of the Rampton Hospital*. (Chairman: Sir John Boynton). London, Her Majesty's Stationery Office.

D.H.S.S. N.I. (1986). *The mental health order.* London, Her Majesty's Stationery Office.

D.H.S.S. N.I. (1986b). *Regional strategy for Northern Ireland..* London, Her Majesty's Stationery Office.

D.H.S.S. (1989). *Working for patients. Government White Paper.* London, Her Majesty's Stationery Office.

D.H.S.S. N.I. (1990). *People first: community care in Northern Ireland in the 1990's.* London, Her Majesty's Stationery Office.

D.H.S.S. N.I. (1987, 1991). *Personal enquiries to statistics and research annexe,* Belfast, DHSS.

D.H.S.S. (1992). *The citizens' charter.* London, Her Majesty's Stationery Office.

D.H.S.S. (1992). *The patients' charter.* London, Her Majesty's Stationery Office.

Dick, J. (1984). *Unpublished report of visiting team to Purdysburn unit of management.* Belfast, Her Majesty's Stationery Office.

Dickoff, J. James, P. (1968). A theory of theories: a position paper. *Nursing Research,* 17(3) :197-203.

Dienemann, J. (1976). The application of psychotherapeutic conceptual models in nursing practice. *Journal Of Psychiatric Nursing and Mental Health Services,* 14(13) :28-30.

Diers, D. (1979). *Research in nursing practice.* Philadelphia, J.B. Lippincott Co.

Donabedian, A. (1966). Evaluating the quality of medical care. *Millbank Memorial Fund Quarterly,* 44(2) :166-206.

Donabedian, A. (1980). *Explorations in quality assessment and monitoring: the d definition of quality and approaches to its assessment.* Ann Arbor, Michican, Health Administration Press.

Draper, P. (1990). The development of theory in British nursing: current position and future prospects. *Journal of Advanced Nursing,* 15 :12-15.

Draper, P. (1991). The ideal and the real: some thoughts on the theoretical developments in British nursing. *Nurse Education Today,* 11 :292-294.

Drummond, J.S. (1990). The work style of students of mental health nursing undertaking the Project 2000 schemes of training: a logical analysis. *Journal of Advanced Nursing,* 15 :977-984.

Dumas, R.G. (1978). Expanding the theoretical framework for effective nursing. *Nursing Clinics of North America,* 13(4) :707-716.

Dyer, S. (1990). Nursing models: teamwork for personal patient care. *Nursing the Elderly,* 1(5) :28-30.

Dykens J.W. Hyde, R.W. Orzack, L.H. York, R.H. (1964). *Strategies of mental hospital change.* Mass, Dept of Mental Health.

Easterbrook, J. ed. (1988). *Care of the elderly.* Choosing a model series. London, Edward Arnold.

234

Eichorn, M.J. Frevert, E.I. (1979). Evaluation of a primary nursing system using the quality of patient care scale. *Journal of Nursing Administration,* 9 :11-13.

Elliott-Cannon, C. (1990). Mental handicap and nursing models. In Salvage, J. Kershaw, B. (eds) *Models for nursing 2.* London, Scutari Press.

Elliott, J.R. (1975). *Living in hospital.* London, King's Fund.

Ellis, R. (1968). Characteristics of significant theories. *Nursing Research,* 17(3) :217-222.

Ellis, R. (1982b). Models of care. *Nursing Mirror,* 155(15) :vii.

Ellis, R. (1982). Conceptual issues in nursing. *Nursing Outlook,* 30(23) :406-410.

Ellsworth, R. Klett, W. Gordon, H. Gunn, R. (1971). Milieu characteristics of successful psychiatric treatment programs. *American Journal of Ortho Psychiatry,* 41(3) :427-441.

Engle, T. Hall, B.A. Mitsunga, B.K. (1978). Social exchange and quality of care on a psychiatric unit. In: *Communitating nursing research.,* Portland, Oregon, W.I.C.H.E. Vol 11.

Engstrom, J.L. (1984). Problems in the development, use and testing of nursitheory. *Journal of Nurse Education,* 23(6) :245-251.

Erickson, R.C. (1975). Outcome studies in mental hospitals: a review. *Psychological Bulletin,* 82 :519-540.

Eysenck, H.J. (1971). A mish-mash of theories. *International Journal of Psychiatry,* 109 :12-18.

Fairweather G.W. Sanders, D. Tornatsky, R. Harris, R. (1974). *Creating change in mental health organisations.* Oxford, Pergamon Press.

Farmer, E. (1986). Exploring the issues. In Kershaw, B. Salvage, J. eds, *Models for nursing.* Chichester, John Wiley & Sons.

Farrell, P. Scherer, K. (1983). The Delphi technique as a method for selecting criteria to evaluate nursing care. *Nursing Papers* (Can), 15(1) :51-60.

Fawcett, J. (1980). A framework for analysis and evaluation of conceptual models of nursing. *Nurse Educator,* 5(12) 12-14.

Fawcett, J. (1984,1989). *Analysis and evaluation of conceptual models of nursing.* Philadelphia, F.A. Davis.

Fawcett, J. Carino, C. (1989). Hallmarks of success in nursing practice. *Advances in Nursing Science,* 11(4) :1-8.

Fawcett, J. (1990). Preparation for Caesarean childbirth: derivation of a nursing intervention from the Roy adaptation model. *Journal of Advanced Nursing,* 15 :1418-1425.

Felton, G. (1975). Increasing the quality of nursing care by introducing the concept of primary nursing: a model project. *Nursing Research,* 24(1) :27-32.

Ferketich, S. (1990). Internal consistency estimates of reliability. *Research in Nursing and Health,* 13 :437-440.

235

Festinger, L. (1964). *Conflict decision and dissonance.* London, Tavistock Publications.

Field, P.A. (1983). An ethnography: four public health nurses' perceptions of nursing. *Journal of Advanced Nursing,* 8 :3-12.

Field, P.A. Morse, J. M. (1985). *Nursing research: the application of qualitative approaches.* London, Croom Helm.

Fifer, W.R. (1980). Quality assurance in health care. In Awad, A.G. Durost, H.B. McCormick, W.Q. (eds). *Evaluation of quality of care in psychiatry.* Toronto, Pergamon Press.

Finch, E. (1986). Professional credibility for the psychiatric nurse: a question of survival. *International Nursing Review,* 33(2) :44-49.

Firlit, S.L. (1990). Nursing theory and nursing practice: do they connect? In McCloskey, G. Grace, H. (eds). *Current Issues in Nursing.* St Louis, C.V. Mosby & Co.

Fitzpatrick, J.J. Whall, A.L. Johnston R.L. Floyd J.A. (1982), *Nursing models: applications to psychiatric mental health nursing.* Maryland, Brady & Co.

Fitzpatrick, J.J. (1982), In, Fitzpatrick, J.J. et al. *Nursing models: application to psychiatric mental health nursing.* Maryland, USA Brady & Co.

Fitzpatrick, J.J. Whall, A.L. (1983,1989). *Conceptual models of nursing: analysis and application.* Norwalk, Conn, Appleton & lange.

Fox, D.J. (1982). *Fundamentals of research in nursing.* 4th ed. Conn, Appleton-Century-Crofts.

Fraser, M. (1990). *Using conceptual nursing in practice: a research based approach.* London, Harper & Row.

Fretwell, J.E. (1978). *Socialisation of nurses: teaching and learning in hospital wards.* University of Warwick, Unpublished Ph.D Thesis.

Fretwell, J.E. (1985). *Freedom to change.* London, Royal College of Nursing.

Freud, S. (1949). *An Outline of psychoanalysis.* New York, W.W. Norton.

Friedrichs, J. (1979). *Methoden empirischer sozialforschung.* Hamburg, Rowohlt :370-373.

Friend, B. (1990). Working at health. *Nursing Times,* 86(16) :21.

Gardner, E. Gardner M. (1971). A community mental health centre: case study, innovations and issues. *Seminars in Psychiatry,* 3(2) :172-198.

Garety, P.A. (1981). *Staff attitudes, organisational structure, and the quality of care of long-stay psychiatric patients.* Institute of Psychiatry, University of London. Unpublished M.Phil.

George, J. Ed, (1985). *Nursing theories, the base for professional practice.* Englewood Cliffs, New Jersey. Prentice Hall,

Georgiades, N.J. Philmore, L. (1976). The myth of the hero innovator and alternative strategies for organisational change. In Kieman, C.C. Woodford, F.P. (eds). *Behaviour modification with the severly retarded.* New York, Scientific Publishers.

Girot, E. (1990). Discussing nursing theory. *Senior Nurse,* 10(6) :16-19.

Glasper, A. (1990). A planned approach to nursing children. In Salvage, J. Kershaw, B. (eds), *Models for Nursing 2*. London, Scutari Press.

Gleit, C. Graham, B. (1989). Secondary data analysis: a valuable resource. *Nursing Research,* 38(6) :380-381.

Goffman, E. (1961). *Asylums: essays on the social situations of mental patients and other inmates*. Middlesex, Pelican.

Goldstone, L. A. Ball, J.A. Collier, M.M. (1983). *Monitor: an index of the quality of nursing care for acute medical and surgical wards*. Newcastle, Newcastle upon Tyne Polytechnic Products Ltd.

Goldstone, L. (1990). *Psychiatric monitor.*. Newcastle, Newcastle Upon Tyne Products Ltd.

Goodman, C.M. (1986). *A Delphi survey of clinical nursing research priorities within a regional health authority*. University of London, Unpub M.Sc Thesis.

Goodman, C.M. (1987). The Delphi technique: a critique. *Journal of Advanced Nursing,* 12 :729-734.

Gordon, D. R. (1984). Research application: identifying the use and misuse of formal models in nursing practice. In Benner, P. (ed) *From novice to expert*, New York, Addison Wesley.

Gottlieb, L. Rowat, K. (1987). The McGill model of nursing: a practice derived model. *Advances in Nursing Science,* 9(4) :51-61.

Gould, D. (1989). Teaching theories and models of nursing: implications for a common foundation programme for nurses. In Akinsanya, J.A. (ed). *Theories and models of nursing*. Edinburgh, Churchill Livingstone.

Grahame, F. (1987). Backchat. *Nursing Times,* 83(16) :22.

Greaves, F. (1984). *Nurse education and the curriculum: a curricular model*. London, Croom Helm :88-93.

Green, C. (1985). An overview of the value of nursing models in relation to education. *Nurse Education Today,* 5 :267-271.

Green, C. (1988). The development of a conceptual model for mental handicap nursing practice in the U.K. *Nurse Education Today,* 8 :9-17.

Griffith, J.W. Christensen, P.J. (1982). *Nursing process, application of theories, frameworks and models*. St Louis, C.V.Mosby.

Griffiths, R. (Chairman) (1984). (HC84 13) *Health service implementation of the NHS Management Enquiry report*. London, HMSO.

Gruenberg, E.M. (1967). The Social breakdown syndrome - some origins. *American Journal of Psychiatry,* 123 :1481-1492.

Grypdonck, M. Koone, G. Rodenback, M. Windy, T. Plain, J.E. (1979). Integrating nursing: a holistic approach to the delivery of nursing care. *International Journal of Nursing Studies,* 16 :215-230.

Guy, M.E. Moore, L.S. (1982). The goal attainment Scale for psychiatric inpatients. *Quality Review Bulletin,* 2(8) :19-29.

237

Hagemeier, D. Hunt, C. (1979). Do new graduates use conceptual frameworks? *Nursing Outlook*, 27 :545-548.

Hale, C. (1991). Evaluating a change to primary nursing: some methodological issues. *Nursing Practice,* 4(4) :12-16.

Halek, C. (1990). Myth or reality?. *Nursing Standard*, 4(37) :47

Hall, K.V. (1979). Current trends in the use of conceptual frameworks in nursing education. *Journal of Nurse Education*, 18(4) :26-29.

Hall, L, (1959). Nursing - what is it? Virginia, *Virginia State Nurses Association,* Winter.

Haller, K.B. Reynolds, M.A. Horsley, J.A. (1979). Developing research based innovation protocols: process criteria, and issues. *Research in Nursing and Health,* 2 :45-51.

Hammill-Cooper, K. (1984). Territorial behaviour among the institutionalised: a nursing perspective. *Journal of Psychosocial Nursing,* 22(12) :6-11.

Hanley, I.G. McGuire, R.J. Boyd, W.D. (1981). Reality orientation and dementia: a controlled trial of two approaches. *British Journal of Psychiatry,* 138 :10-14.

Hardy, L.K. (1982). Nursing models and research - a restricting view? *Journal of Advanced Nursing*, 7 :447-451.

Hardy, L.K. (1986). Janforum. Identifying the place of theoretical frameworks in an evolving discipline. *Journal of Advanced Nursing*, 11 :103-107.

Hargie, O. McCartan, P.J. (1986). *Social skills training and psychiatric nursing.* London, Croom Helm.

Harre, R. (1972). *The philosophies of science: an introductory survey.* Oxford, Oxford University Press.

Hawkett, S. (1989). A model marriage. *Nursing Times*, 85(1) :61-62.

Hays, J. (1975). cited in Huey, F.L. *Psychiatric nursing 1946-1974: a report of the state of the art.* New York, American Journal of Nursing Co :28.

Hayward, J. (1975). *Information - a prescription against pain.* London, Royal College of Nursing.

Henderson, C. (1990). Models and midwifery. In Salvage, J. and Kershaw, B. (eds). *Models for nursing 2.* London, Scutari press.

Henderson, V. Harmer, B. (1955). *Textbook of the principles and practices of nursing.* 5th ed. New York, Macmillan.

Henderson, V. (1966). *The nature of nursing: a definition and its implications for practice, education and research.* London, Collier Macmillan.

Herbert, M. (1988). The value of nursing models. *The Canadian Nurse,* 84(12) :32-34.

Hersey, P. Blanchard, K.H. (1977). *Management of organisational behaviour.* New Jersey, Prentice Hall.

Herzberg, F. (1968). *Work and the nature of man.* London, Staples Press.

Hitch, P.J. Murgatroyd, J.D. (1983). Professional communications in cancer care: a Delphi survey of hospital nurses. *Journal of Advanced Nursing*, 8 :413-422.

Hjorten, M.K. (1982). A volunteer support system for the chronically mentally ill. *Perspectives in Psychiatric Care,* XX(1) :17-22.

Hoch, C.C. (1987). Assessing delivery of nursing care. *Journal of Gerontological Nursing,* 13(1) :10-17.

Hockey, L. (1982). Some methodological issues in nursing research. In Redfern, S (ed), *Issues in Nursing Research.* Macmillan Press, London.

Hofford, E.C. (1976). Standards of nursing care. *Nursing Times,* 72 :1439-1442.

Holden, R.J. (1990). Models, muddles and medicine. *International Journal of Nursing Studies,* 27(3) :223-234.

Hollingsworth, C. (1985). *Preparation for change.* London, Royal College of Nursing.

Honigfeld, G. Klett, R.D. (1965). The nurses observation scale for inpatient evaluation: a new scale for measuring improvement in chronic schizophrenia. *Journal of Clinical Psychology,* 21 :65-71.

Houlihan, P.J. (1986). The Marketing of nursing jargon. *The Canadian Nurse.* 82(21) :21-22.

Hume, C. Pullan, I. (1986). *Rehabilitation in psychiatry: an ntroductory handbook.* Edinburgh, Churchill Livingstone.

Humphries, G.M. Turner, A. (1989). Job satisfaction and attitudes of nursing staff on a unit for the elderly severely mentally infirm, with change of location. *Journal of Advanced Nursing,* 14 :298-307.

Hurst, K. (1988). Patient satisfaction in outpatients. *Nursing Times,* 84(50) :47.

Ironbar, N. Okon (1985) *Self instruction in psychiatric nursing.* London, Bailliere Tindall.

Jackson, M. (1986). On maps and models. *Senior Nurse,* 5(4) :24-26.

Jacobson, S. (1987). Studying and using conceptual models of nursing. *Image,* 19(2) :78-83.

Jacox, A. (1974). Theory construction in nursing: an overview. *Nursing Research,* 32(1) :4-13.

Jennings, B.M. Meleis, A.I. (1988). Nursing theory and administrative practice. *Advances in Nursing Science,* 10(3) :56-69.

Johns, C. (1990). Developing a philosophy. *Nursing Practice,* 4(1) :2-6.

Johnson, D.E. (1959). The Nature of a science of nursing. *Nursing Outlook,* 7 :291-294.

Johnson, M. (1983). Some aspects of the relation between theory and research in nursing. *Journal of Advanced Nursing,* 8 :21-28.

Johnson, M.B. (1990). The holistic paradigm in nursing: the diffusion of an innovation. *Research in Nursing and Health,* 13 :129-139.

239

Jones, M. (1953). *The therapeutic community: a new treatment method in psychiatry.* New York, Basic Books.

Jones, W.L. (1983). *Ministering to minds diseased. A history of psychiatric treatment.* London, Heinemann Ltd.

Jones, C.M.W. (1987). *Social atmosphere on acute hospital wards as perceived by patients and staff.* University of Manchester, Unpublished M.Sc Thesis.

Jones, R.G. (1988). Experimental study to evaluate nursing staff morale in a high stimulation geriatric psychiatry setting. *Journal of Advanced Nursing,* 13 :352-357.

Jones, A. (1990). The value of models in district nursing. In: Salvage, J. Kershaw, B. (eds). *Models for nursing 2.* London, Scutari Press.

Judson, H.F. (1980). *The search for solutions.* New York, Holt, Rinehart and Wilson.

Jukes, M. (1988). Nursing model or psychological assessment? *Senior Nurse,* 8(11) :8-10.

Kasch, C.R. (1986). Towards a theory of nursing action: skills and competency in nurse-patient interaction. *NursingResearch,* 35(4) :226-230.

Keddie, A.C. (1978). *The Influence of dayroom seating arrangement on behaviour in a psychiatric hospital ward.* University of Exeter, Unpublished M.Sc. Thesis.

Kemp, V.A. (1990). Themes in theory development. In Chaska, N.L. (ed). *The nursing profession: turning points.* St Louis, C.V. Mosby & Co.

Kent, L.A. (1978, 1983). *Outcomes of a comparative study of primary, team, and case methods of nursing care delivery in terms of quality of patient care and staff satisfaction in six Western Region hospitals.* Primary Nursing Research Group, Oregon, WICHE.

Kent, J. Barnett, B. Koster, A. Owen, K. Palmer, S. Phillips, N. Vernon, S. (1990). *Research with not on...challenging the scientific model.* Cardiff, Paper presented at the RCN Annual Research Conference.

Kershaw, B. Salvage, J. (eds) (1986). *Models for nursing.* Chichester, John Wiley & Sons.

Kershaw, B. (1986). Introduction. In Kershaw, B. Salvage, J.(eds). *Models for nursing.* Chichester, John Wiley & Sons.

Kershaw, B. (1990). Towards 2000. In Salvage, J. Kershaw, B. (eds) *Models for nursing 2.* London, Scutari Press.

Kershaw, B. (1990b). Nursing models as philosophies of care. *Nursing Practice,* 4(1) :25-28.

Kesey K. (1962). *One flew over the cuckoo's nest.* London, Pan Books Ltd.

Keyzer, D.M. (1985). *Learning contracts: the trained nurse and the implementation of the nursing process: comparative case studies in the management of knowledge and change in nursing practice.* Institute of Education, University of London, Unpublished Ph.D thesis.

Kim, H.S. (1983). *The Nuture of theoretical thinking in nursing.* Norwalk, Conn, Appleton-Century-Crofts.

King, I. (1968), A conceptual frame of reference for nursing. *Nursing Research,* 17(1) :27-31.

Kinlein, M.L. (1977). The self care concept. *American Journal of Nursing,* 77 :598-601.

Kitson A L & Kendall H (1986) Quality assurance. *Nursing Times,* 82(35) 29-31.

Kitson A L, Hyndman S J, Harvey G, Yerrell P (1990) *Quality patient care, an introduction to RCN dynamic standard setting system (DySSSy)*, London, Scutari.

Knapp, T.R. (1990). Treating ordinal scales as interval scales: an attempt to resolve the controversy. *Nursing Research,* 39(2) :121-123.

Kramer, M. (1974). *Reality shock: why nurses leave nursing.* St Louis, C.V. Mosby & Co.

Kristjanson, L.J. Tamblyn, R. Kuypers, J.A.(1987). A model to guide development and application of multiple nursing theories. *Journal of Advanced Nursing,* 12 :523-529.

Kuhn, T. (1970). *The structure of scientific revolution.* Chicago, University of Chicago Press.

Lamb, H.R. (1979). Staff burnout in work with long-term patients. *Hospital and Community Psychiatry,* 30(6) :396-398.

LaMonica, E.L. Oberst, M.T. Madea, A.R. Wolf, R.M. (1986). Development of a patient satisfaction scale. *Research in Nursing and Health,* 9 :43-50.

Lancaster, J. (1979). Community treatment for mental health's forgotton population. *Journal of Psychiatric Nursing and Mental Health Services,* 17(4) :20-27.

Lancaster, J. Lancaster, W. (1982). *The nurse as a change agent.* St Louis, C.V Mosby & Co.

Lundewcerd, J.A. Doumans, N.P.G. (1988). Nurses' work satisfaction and feelings of health and stress in three psychiatric departments. *International Journal of Nursing Studies,* 25(3) :225-234.

Lane, D.E. (1983). Institutional care. In. Adams, C.G. Macione, A. eds. *Handbook of psychiatric mental health nursing.* New York, John Wiley & Sons.

Lang, N. (1974). *A model for quality assurance in nursing.* University of Milwaulkie Winsconsin, Unpublished Ph.D Thesis.

Lau, G. (1990). Closing time. *Nursing Times,* 86(22) :40-41.

Leddy, S. Pepper, J.M. (1989). *Conceptual bases of professional nursing.* Philadelphia, J.B. Lippincott Co.

Lego, S. (1975). The one to one nurse-patient relationship. In Huey, F.L. *Psychiatric nursing 1946-1974: a report of the state of the art.* New York, American Journal of Nursing Co.

241

Leininger, M.M. (1978). *Transcultural nursing: concepts, theories and practices*. New York, John Wiley & Sons.

Lemmer, B. Smits, M. (1989). *Facilitating change in mental health*. London, Chapman & Hall.

Lerheim, K. (1991). Nursing science - does it make a difference? *International Nursing Review*, 38(3) :73-78.

Levine, M.E. (1966). Adaptation and assessment: a rationale for nursing intervention. *American Journal of Nursing*, 66(11) :2450-2453.

Lewin, K. (1946). Action research and minority problems. *Journal of Social Issues*, 2 :34-46.

Lewin, K. (1951). *Field theory in social science*. Conn, Greenwood Press.

Limieux-Charles, L. (1980). *Blueprint for nursing*. Toronto, College of Nurses of Ontario.

Lindeman, C.A. (1975). Delphi survey of priorities in clinical nursing research. *Nursing Research*, 24(6) :434-441.

Lindsay, B. (1990). The gap between theory and practice. *Nursing Standard*, 5(4) :34-35.

Linn, L. (1970). State hospital environment and rates of patient discharge. *Archives of General Psychiatry,* 23 :346-351.

Linstone, H.A. Turoff, M. (1975). *The Delphi method: techniques and applications*. Reading, Mass, Addison-Wesley Publ Co inc.

Lippitt, G (1973). *Visualising change: model building and the change process*. La Jolla, Calif, University Associates Inc.

Lister, P. (1987). The Misunderstood model. *Nursing Times*, 83(41) :40-42.

Littlewood, J (1989). A model for nursing using anthropological literature. *International Journal of Nursing Studies*, 26(3) :221-229.

Longhorn, E. (1984) *Psychiatric care and conditions*. 2nd ed. Chichester, John Wiley & Sons.

Loughlin, K.G. Moore, L.F. (1979). Using delphi to achieve congruent objectives and activities in a peadiatrics department. *Journal of Medical Education,* 54(2) :101-106.

Loughlin, M. (1988). Modelled, muddled and befuddled. *Nursing Times,* 84(5) :30-31.

Luft, S. (1990). Measuring patient dependency. *Nursing,* 4(9) 13-16.

Luker, K. (1987). *Applying models of nursing in the community*. London, Paper read at 2nd International Primary Health Care Conference.

Luker, K. (1988). Debate 1. This house believes that nursing models provide a useful tool in the management of patient care. In Pritchard, A.P. (ed) *Proceedings of the 5th International Conference on Cancer Nursing*, London, Macmillan Press.

Lyons, H. (1981). Solutions by consensus. *Health and Social Services Journal*, XCL :1515-1516.

MacIlwaine, H. (1980). *The nursing care of neurotic patients in psychiatric units of a general hospital*. University of Manchester, Unpublished Ph.D. Thesis.

MacMillan, M (1989). *A Delphi survey of priorities for nursing research in Scotland*. Edinburgh, Department of Nursing Studies.

Macleod Clark, J. Hockey, L. (1979). *Research for nursing: a guide for the enquiring nurse*. London, H, M & M Publishers.

McClune, B.A. (1986). *Job satisfaction and dissatisfaction of nurses on a general/ cardio thoracic intensive care unit*. University of Surrey, Unpublished M.Sc Thesis.

McClymont, M.E. (1985) Intervention and care in long-term nursing of the adult. In, King, K. ed. *Recent advances in nursing 13. Long term care*. Edinburgh, Churchill Livingstone.

McFarlane, J.K. (1977). Developing a theory of nursing: the relation of theory to practice, education, and research. *Journal of Advanced Nursing*, 2 :261-270.

McFarlane, J.K. (1982). *Nursing: a paradigm of caring.Ethical issues in caring*. University of Manchester, Unpublished Paper.

McFarlane, J.K. (1986). Looking to the future. In, Kershaw, B. Salvage, J. eds. *Models for nursing*. Chichester, John Wiley & Sons.

MacGuire, J. Botting, D.A. (1990). The use of the Ethnograph program to identify the perceptions of nursing staff following the introduction of primary nursing in an acute medical ward for elderly people. *Journal of Advanced Nursing*, 15 :1120-1127.

McGhee, A. (1961). *The patient's attitude to nursing care*. Edinburgh, Churchill Livingstone.

McGilloway, F.A.(1981). In Smith, J.P. ed. *Nursing science in nursing practice*. London, Butterworths.

McGregor, D. (1960). *The human side of enterprise*. New York, McGraw Hill.

McKenna, H.P. (1989). The selection by ward managers of an appropriate nursing model for long-stay psychiatric patient care. *Journal of Advanced Nursing*, 14 :762-775.

Maloney, E. (1984). Theoretical approaches. In, Beck, C.A. Rawlings, R.P. Williams,S.R. *Mental health psychiatric nursing: a holistic life cycle approach*. St Louis, C.V. Mosby & Co.

Mansfield, E. (1980). A conceptual framework for psychiatric mental health care nursing. *Journal of Psychiatric Nursing and Mental Health Services* 18(4):34-41.

Manthey, M. Ciske, K. Robertson, P. (1970). Primary nursing. *Nursing Forum*, 9(1) :64-83.

Manthey, M. (1980). *The practice of primary nursing*. Boston, Blackwell Publications.

Marks, I.M. Hallam, R.S. Connolly, J. Philpott, R. (1977). *Nursing in behavioural psychotherapy*. London, Royal College of Nursing.

243

Marks, I.M. (1985). *Psychiatric nurse therapists in primary care*. London, Royal College of Nursing.

Marks, I.M. (1986). *Behaviour psychotherapy: Maudsley pocket book of clinical management*. Bristol, Wright.

Marram, G. Flynn, K. Abaravich, W. Carey, S. (1976). *Cost effectiveness of primary and team nursing*. Wakefield, Mass, Contemporary Publishing Inc.

Marshall, R. Bilbe, M. (1990). Sweeping assumptions away. *Nursing Times*, 86(18) :36-38.

Martin, E. (1974). *Hospitals in trouble*. Oxford, Blackwell Press.

Martin, E. J.(1985). A Specialty in decline? psychiatric mental health nursing, past, present and future. *Journal of Professional Nursing,* 1(1) :48-53.

Martin, L. Glasper, A. (1986). Core plans: nursing models and the nursing process in action. *Nursing Practice*, 1 :268-273.

Martin, M.L. Kirkpatrick, H. (1987). *Nursing conceptual frameworks: do nurses find them useful in practice?* Edinburgh, Poster Presentation at International Research Conference.

Maslow, A.H. (1954). *Motivation and personality.* New York, Harper & Row.

Mason, T. Chanley, M. (1990). Nursing models in a special hospital: a critical analysis of efficacity. *Journal of Advanced Nursing*, 15 :667-673.

Mauksch, I.G. Miller, M.H. (1981). *Implementing change in nursing*. St Louis, C.V. Mosby & Co.

Meenz, G. (1988). *Psychiatric monitor, Vol 2: long-stay/ continuing care*. Birmingham, North West Nurse Staffing Levels Project. International Health Services Ltd.

Meleis, A.I. (1985). *Theoretical nursing: development and progress*. Philadelphia, J.B. Lippincott.

Melia, K. (1990). Nursing models: enhancing or inhibiting practice? *Nursing Standard*, 5(11) :34-35.

Menzies, I.E.P. (1960). A case study in the functioning of social systems as a defense against anxiety: A report of a study of the nursing service of a general hospital. *Human Relations*, 13(2) :95-121.

Merchant, J. (1991). Task allocation: a case of resistance to change. *Nursing Practice*, 4(2) :16-18.

Mercier, C. (1986). Intervention in the psychiatric hospital in the Era of deinstitu -tionalisation. *Canada's Mental Health,* 34(3) :13-17.

Merton, R.K. (1968). *Social theory and social structure.* New York, Free Press.

Metcalf, C. (1982). *A Study of a change in the method of organising the delivery of Nursing Care in a ward of a Maternity Hospital*. University Of Manchester, Unpublished D.Phil Thesis.

Meyer, J. (1992). *The trials and tribulations of action research.* University of Birmingham, Paper presented at the Royal College of Nursing's Research Advisory Group Annual Conference.

Midgley, C. (1988). *The use of models for nursing within midwifery training hospitals in England.* Huddersfield Polytechnic, Huddersfield, Unpublished paper.

Miller, A.E. (1985). The relationship between nursing theory and nursing practice. *Journal of Advanced Nursing,* 10 :414-424.

Miller, A.E. (1989). Theory to practice: implementing in the clinical setting. In Jolly, M. Allen, P. (eds). *Current issues in nursing.* London, Chapman Hall.

Miller, A.E. (1989b). *A study of work organisation by nurses in relation to patient outcomes in geriatric hospital wards.* University of Manchester, Unpublished Ph.D Thesis.

Milne, D. (1986). Planning and evaluating innovations in nursing practice by measuring the ward atmosphere. *Journal of Advanced Nursing,* 11 :203 - 210.

MIND, (1975). *Report: mental health statistics.* London, MIND.

MIND, (1977). *Better prospects: rehabilitation in mental illness hospitals. A report on facilities in 84 hospitals.* London, MIND.

Ministry of Health. (1968). *Psychiatric nursing: today and tomorrow.* London, Her Majesty's Stationary Office.

Minshull, J. Ross, K. Turner, J. (1986). The human needs model of nursing. *Journal of Advanced Nursing,* 11 :643-649.

Mirabi, M. Winman, M.L. Magnetti, S.M. Keppler, K.M. (1985). Professional attitudes towards the chronic mentally ill. *Hospital and Community Psychiatry,* 36(4) :404-405.

Mitchell, B. Hughes, J. (1980). Psychiatric nursing - what future? *Nursing Focus.* 1(6) :234-237.

Moos, R.H. (1974). *Evaluating treatment environments: a socioecological approach.* London, J. Wiley & Sons.

Morse, J.M. (1991). Approaches to qualitative - quantitative methodological triangulation. *Nursing Research,* 40(1) :120-123.

Moscow, D. (1986). Effective implementation of organisational development in the NHS. *Health Services Manpower Review,* 12(2) :3-7.

Murgatroyd, J. Hitch, P. (1984). Professional problems investigated. *Nursing Mirror,* 159(4) :36-37.

Murphy, J.F. (1971). *Theoretical issues in professional nursing.* New York, John Wiley & Sons.

Nachmias, C. Nachmias, D. (1981). *Research methods in the social sciences.* 2nd ed. New York, St Martin's Press.

Neuman, B. Young, R.J. (1972,1982). A model for teaching total person approach to patient problems. *Nursing Research,* 21(3) :264.

Newman, M.A. (1979). *Theory development in nursing.* Philadelphia, F.A. Davis & Co.

Nie, N. Hull, C. Jenkins J. (1970). *Statistical package for the social sciences.* 2nd ed. New York, McGraw Hill.

Nightingale, F. (1859.1980). *Notes on nursing: what it is and what it is not.* Edinburgh, Churchill Livingstone.

NINB (1987). *Report of the inspection of clinical facilities* Belfast, Northern Ireland National Board for Nurses, Midwives and Health Visitors.

Nodder, T.E. (1980). *Organisation and management: problems of mental illness hospitals, report of a working group.* London, Her Majesty's Stationery Office.

Nolan, P.W. (1985). Psychiatry under fire. *Nursing Mirror,* 160 (21) :34-37.

Nolan, P.W. (1989). *Psychiatric nursing past and present: the nurses' viewpoint.* University of Bath, Unpublished Ph.D Thesis.

Norusis, M.J. (1988). *The SPSS guide to data analysis for SPSS/PC+,* Chicago, SPSS Inc.

NPEWG (1986). *Report of the nursing process evaluation working group.* London, Nursing Research Unit, King's College, University of London.

N U P R D (1989). *Patients needs survey.* London, National Unit for Psychiatric Research and Development.

Nursing Theories Conference Group,(1975,1985) *Nursing theories: the base for professional practice* (Chairman, Julia George), New Jersey, Prentice Hall.

Nursing Times, (1989). Editorial. *Nursing Times* 85(27) :3.

Oberst, M. (1978). Priorities in cancer nursing research.*Cancer Nursing,* 1(4) :281-290.

O'Brien, D. Clinton, M. Cruddace, H. (1985). *Managing and mismanaging change: the case of the nursing process.* Newcastle-upon-Tyne, The educational development unit.

O'Neill, J.E. (1984). *The use of nursing records in the evaluation of nursing care.* University of Manchester, Unpublished M.Sc Thesis.

Openshaw, S. (1984). *Clinical judgement by nurses: decision strategies and nurses' appraisal of patient affect.* University of London, Unpublished Ph.D Thesis.

Orem, D.E. (1958, 1980). *Nursing: concepts of practice.* New York, McGraw Hill.

Orlando, I.J. (1961). *The dynamic nurse-patient relationship* New York, G.P. Putnam.

Ottoway, R.N. (1976). A change strategy to implement new norms, new style and new environment in the work organisation. *Personnel Review,* 5(1) :13-18.

Oxford Dictionary of Quotations. (1988). 3rd edition. London, Guild Publications.

Parahoo, K. (1991). Job satisfaction of community psychiatric nurses in Northern Ireland. *Journal of Advanced Nursing,* 16 :317-324.

Parse, R.R. (1981). *Man-living-health: a theory of nursing.* New York, John Wiley & Sons.

Parsons, T. (1952). *The social system.* London, Tavistock Publications.

Patterson, J.G. Zderad, L.T. (1976). *Humanistic nursing.* New York, John Wiley & Sons.

Pavlov, I.P. (1927). *Conditioned reflexes: an investigation of the physiological activity of the cerebral cortex*. London, Oxford University Press.

Paykel, E.S. Mangen, S.P. Griffiths, J.H. Burns, T.P. (1982). Community psychiatric nursing for neurotic patients: a controlled trial. *British Journal of Psychiatry*, 140 :573-581.

Pearson, A. (1985). Nurses as change agents and a strategy for change. *Nursing Practice*, 2 :80-84.

Pearson, A. (1985b). *The effects of introducing new norms in a nursing unit and an analysis of the process of change*. University of London, Unpublished Ph.D thesis.

Pearson, A. (1986). Nursing models and multidisciplinary teamwork. In, Kershaw, B. Salvage, J. eds. *Models for nursing*. Chichester, John Wiley & Sons.

Pearson, A. Vaughan, B. (1986). *Nursing models for practice*. London, Heinemann.

Peplau, H.E. (1952). *Interpersonal relations in nursing*. New York, G.P.Putnam & Sons.

Perkins, (1965). Cited in Hoon, E. (1986). Game playing: a new way to look at models. *Journal of Advanced Nursing*, 11 :421-427.

Phaneuf, M.C. (1966). The nursing audit for evaluation of patient care. *Nursing Outlook*, 14 :51-54.

Philip, A.E. (1973). A note on the nurses' observation scale for inpatient evaluation (NOSIE). *British Journal of Psychiatry*, 122 :595-596.

Philip, A.E. (1977). Cross-culteral study of the factorial dimensions of the NOSIE. *Journal of Clinical Psychology*, 33(2) :467-468.

Phillips, L.R.F. (1986). *A clinicians guide to the critique and utilisation of nursing research*. Norwalk, Conn, Appleton-Century-Crofts.

Pines, A. Maslach, C. (1978). Characteristics of staff burnout in mental health settings. *Hospital and Community Psychiatry*, 29 :233-237.

Polit, D.F. Hungler, B.P. (1987). *Nursing research: principles and methods*. 3rd ed. Philadelphia, J.B. Lippincott Co.

Powell, D. (1982). *Learning to relate*. Lndon, Royal College of Nursing.

Procter, S. (1985). *The development of a method of incorporating into the nursing service manpower planning system the effects on the provision of nursing produced by the dual status of nurse learners as trainees and employees*. Polytech of The South Bank, London, Unpublished Ph.D Thesis.

Procter, S. (1989). The functioning of nursing routines in the management of a transient workforce. *Journal of Advanced Nursing*, 14(3) :180-189.

Pullan, I.(1986). Historical introduction. In Hume, C. Pullan, I. eds. *Rehabilitation in psychiatry: an introductory handbook*. Edinburgh, Churchill Livingstone.

Raphael, W. (1978). *Psychiatric hospitals viewed by their patients*. London, King'sFund.

Rapoport, R. (1960). *Community as doctor: new perspectives on a therapeutic community*. London, Tavistock Publications.

Rauch, W. (1979). The decision Delphi. *Technological Forecasting and Social Change*, 15 :159-169.

Rawnsley, K. (1986). Summing up. In Wilkinson, G. Freeman, H. eds. *The provision of mental health services in Britain: the way ahead*. London, Gaskell.

Reason, P. (ed) (1988). *Human enquiry in action*. London, Sage Publications.

Redfern, S. J. & Norman, I. J. (1990). Measuring the quality of nursing care: a consideration of different approaches. *Journal of Advanced Nursing* 15 :1260-1271.

Reed, J. Robbins, I (1991). Models of nursing: their relevance to the care of elderly people. *Journal of Advanced Nursing*, 16 :1350-1357.

Reed, P.G. (1987). Constructing a conceptual framework for psychosocial nursing. *Journal of Psyhosocial Nursing*, 25(2) :24-28.

Reid, N.G. (1985). *Wards in chancery*? London, Royal College of Nursing.

Reid, N.G. (1988). The Delphi technique, its contribution to the evaluation of professional practice. In Ellis, R. (ed). *Professional competence and quality assurance in the caring professions*. London, Croom Helm.

Reid, N.G. Boore J.R.P. (1987). *Research methods and statistics in health care*. London, Edward Arnold.

Reilly, D.E. (1975). Why a conceptual framework? *Nursing Outlook*, 23(9) :566-569.

Reimer, T.T. (1985). Combining qualitative and quantitative methodologies. In Leininger, M.M. (ed) *Qualitative research methods in nursing*. Orlando, Grune and Stratton.

Reinkemeyer, A.M. (1970). Commitment to an ideology of change. *Nursing Forum*, lX(2) :340-355.

Rhodes, B. (1985). *An investigation into the usefulness of a theoretical decision making model of nursing*. University of Leeds, Unpublished Ph.D. thesis.

Riehl, J.P. (1974). The Riehl interactional model. In, Riehl, J.P. Roy, C. eds *Conceptual models in nursing practice*. New York, Appleton-Century-Crofts.

Riehl, J.P. Roy, C.(1974,1980). *Conceptual models for nursing practice*. New York, Appleton-Century-Crofts.

Robinson, K. (1990). Nursing models: the hidden costs. *Surgical Nurse*, 3(7) :11-14.

Rogers, E. (1983). *Diffusion of innovations*. New York, Free Press.

Rogers, J.A. (1974). Theoretical considerations involved in the process of change. In Backer, B.A. Dubbert, P.M. Eisenman, E.J.P. (eds) *Psychiatric/mental health nursing: contemporary readings*. New York, D.Van Nostrand Co Ltd.

Rogers, M.E. (1970). *An introduction to a theoretical basis of nursing*. Philadelphia, F.A. Davis & Co.

Rogers, R. (1986). Choosing is taking a political stance. *Senior Nurse*, 5(4) :4

Roosevelt, T. (1913). cited in: The Oxford dictionary of quotations. 3rd edition. London, Guild Publishers.

Roper, N. Logan, W. Tierney, A. (1983). *Using a model for nursing*. Edinburgh, Churchill Livingstone.

Roper, N. Logan, N. Tierney, A. (1980,1985,1990). *Elements of nursing*, (1st, 2nd & 3rd ed). Edinburgh, Churchill Livingstone.

Rosenbaum, J.N. (1986). Comparison of two theorists on Care: Orem and Leininger. *Journal of Advanced Nursing*, 11 :409-419.

Ross, T. (1981). Thought control. psychiatry 5. *Nursing Mirror*, 156(21) :16-19.

Rottor, J.B. (1966). Generalised expectancies for internal versus external control of reinforcement. *Psychological Monographs*, 80(1) :19-24.

Roy, C. (1970). Adaptation - a conceptual framework for nursing. *Nursing Outlook*, 18(3) :42-45.

Roy, C. (1971). Adaptation: a basis for nursing practice. *Nursing Outlook*, 19(4) :254-257.

Roy, C. (1980). The Roy adaptation model. In. Riehl, J.P. Roy, C.(eds). *Conceptual models for nursing practice*. New York, Appleton-Century-Crofts.

Rosendal, N. (1983). Maladaptive patterns of response: the chronic client. In Adams, C.G. Macione, A. eds, *Handbook of psychiatric mental health nursing*. New York, John Wiley & Sons.

Rubin, A. Johnson, P.J. (1982). Practitioner orientations toward the chronically disabled: prospects for policy implementation. *Administration Mental Health*, 10(1) :3-12.

Sackman, H. (1975). *Delphi critique*. Lexington, Mass, Lexington Books.

Salanders, L. Dietz Omar, M. (1991). Making nursing models relevant for the pacticing nurse. *Nursing Practice*, 4(2) :23-25.

Salvage, J. (1985). *The politics of nursing*. London, Heinemann.

Salvage, J. (1986). Models to move nursing forward. (News), *Senior Nurse*, 5(4) :4.

Salvage, J. (1990). Introduction. In Salvage, J. Kerehaw, B. (eds). *Models of Nursing2*. London, Scutari Press.

Salvage, J. Kershaw, B. (1990). *Models for nursing 2*. London, Scutari Press.

Sampson, E. (1971). *Social psychology and contemporary science*. New York, John Wiley & Sons.

Scan. (1987). Purdysburn new unit officially opened. *Scan*, 6(39) :1

Schein, E.H. (1969). *Organisational psychology*. New Jersey, Prentice Hall.

Scherer, K. Cameron, C. Farrell, P. (1982). *Summary report: responses to the delphi survey to validate the Manitoba Association of Regisered Nurses standards of nursing care*. Victoria, Canada, Proceedings of the Nursing Research Conference.

Schmieding, T. (1990). An integrative nursing theoretical framework. *Journal of Advanced Nursing*, 15 :463-467.

Schuler, S. Campbell, L.B. (1974). The theme is change. In Backer, B.A. Dubbert, P.M. Eisenman, E.J.P. (eds) *Psychiatric/mental health nursing: contemporary readings*, New York, D.Van Nostrand Co Ltd.

Seligman, M. (1971). Fall into helplessness. *Psychology Today,* 7 :43-48.

Sharp, T. (1991). Whose problem? *Nursing Times,* 87(3) :36-38.

Shepherd, G. (1984). *Institutional care and rehabilitation.* London, Longman.

Siegal, J. (1980). Physical environmental stresses. In Gibbs, M.S. Lachenmeyer, R.J. Siegal, J. eds. *Community psychology.* New York, Gardner Press.

Siegal, S. Castellan, N.J. (1988). *Nonparametric statistics for the behavioural sciences.* 2nd ed. London, McGraw-Hill.

Siegler, M. Osmond, H. (1974). *Models of madness, models of medicine.* New York, Macmillan Publishing Co Inc.

Silva, M. (1977). Philosophy, science, theory: interrelationships and implications for nursing research. *Image,* 9(3) :59-63.

Silva, M.C. (1986). Research testing nursing theory: the state of the art. *Advances in Nursing Science,* 9(1) :1-11.

Sims, J. (1989). The patients' bank. *Nursing Times,* 85(3) :20.

Skinner, B.F. (1938). *The Behaviour of organisms: an experimental analysis.* New York, Appleton-Century-Crofts.

Smith, L. (1986). Issues raised by the use of nursing models in psychiatry. *Nurse Education Today,* 6, :69-75.

Smith, L. (1987). Applications of a nursing model to a curriculum: some considerations. *Nurse Education Today,* 7 :109-115.

Smoyak, S. (1988). *Knowledge is knowledge.* Paper presented at the Fifth Nursing Science Colloquium, Boston, Mass, Boston University School of Nursing.

Sorensen, K.C. Luckmann, J. (1986). *Basic nursing: a psychophysiologic approach.* 2nd ed. Philadelphia, W.B. Saunders Co :159-205.

South East Thames Regional Health Authority (1976). *Report of the committee of enquiry, St Augustines Hospital,* London, Chartham.

Sternberg, P. (1986). Models and theories have not changed practice. (Letter), *Nursing Times,* 83(46) :12.

Stevens, B.J. (1979). *Nursing theory: analysis, application, evaluation.* Boston, Little, Brown & Co.

Stevens, B. (1981). Nursing theories: one or many. In, McCloskey, J.C. Grace, H.K. eds. *Current issues in nursing.* Boston, Blackwell.

Storch, JL (1986) In defence of nursing theory. *The Canadian Nurse.* 82(16) :16-20.

Stockwell, F. (1985). *The nursing process in Psychiatric Nursing.* London, Croom Helm.

Strauss, H.J. Ziegler, L.H. (1975). The Delphi technique and its uses in social science research. *Journal of Creative Behaviour,* 9(4) :253-259.

Street C.G. (1986). An investigation of the priority on nurse-patient interaction by psychiatric nurses. In Brooking, J. ed. *Psychiatric nursing research.* Chichester, John Wiley & Sons.

Stuart, G.W. Sundeen, S.J. (1983). *Principles and practices of psychiatric nursing*. St Louis, C.V. Mosby & Co :32-60.

Suchman, E.A. (1967). *Evaluative research*. New York, Russell Sage Foundation.

Sugden. J. (1977). The psychiatric treatment setting: some general consideration. In Altschul, A. Simpson, R (eds) *Issues in psychiatric nursing*. London, Balliere Tindall.

Sullivan, G.C. (1989). Evaluating Antonovsky's salutogenic model for its adaptability to nursing. *Journal of advanced nursing*. 14 :336-342.

Sullivan, H. (1953). *The Interpersonal theory of psychiatry*. New York, W.W. Norton.

Sumner, E.C. (1981). Psychiatric nursing: the quiet revolution. *Nursing*. 5 :1333-35.

Suppe, F. Jacox, A. (1985). Philosophy of science and the development of nursing theory, In, Werley, H. Fitzpatrick, J.J. (eds), *Annual Review of Nursing Research*, 3 :241-267.

Susman, G.I. Everad, R.D. (1978). An assessment of the scientific merits of action research. *Administrative Science Quarterly*, 23 :582-603.

Sutton, G. (1981). The organisation and administration of nursing services for long-stay patients, In, Wing, J.K. Morris, B. eds. *Handbook of psychiatric rehabilitation practice*. Oxford, Oxford University Press.

Szasz, T. (1961). *The myth of mental illness*. New York, Hoeber-Harper.

Thibodeau, J.A. (1983), *Nursing models: analysis and evaluation*. Monterey, Calif, Wadsworth Health Services Division.

Thomas, L. (1983) *The youngest science: notes of a medicine watcher*. New York, Viking Press :67.

Tierney, A. (1973). Toilet training. *Nursing Times*, 69 :1740-1745.

Tissier, J.M. (1986). The development of a psychiatric nursing assessment form. In Brooking, J. ed. *Psychiatric nursing research*. Chichester, John Wiley & Sons.

Toews, J. Barnes, G. (1986). The Chronic mental patient and community psychiatry: a system in trouble. *Canada's Mental Health*, 34(2) :2-7.

Toffler, A. (1970). *Future shock*. New York, Random House Publ.

Tomlinson, D. (1991). Seeing patients through. *Nursing Times*, 87(8) :54-56.

Torres, G. Yura, N. (1974). *Today's conceptual framework: its relationship to the curriculum development process*. Pub. No. 15-1529. New York, National League of Nursing.

Tosses, G. (1989). *Theoretical foundations of nursing*. Norwalk, Conn, Appleton-Century-Crofts.

Towell, D. (1975). *Understanding psychiatric nursing*. London, Royal College of Nursing.

Towell, D. Harries, C. (eds) (1979). *Innovation in patient care*. London, Croom Helm.

Travelbee, J. (1966). *Interpersonal aspects of nursing*. Philadelphia, F.A. Davis.

Treece, E.W. Treece, J.W. (1977). *Elements of research in nursing*. St Louis, C.V. Mosby & Co.

Turner, J. (1990). *Personal correspondance.*

Turoff, M. (1970). The design of a policy Delphi. *Technological Forecasting and Social Change*, 2(2) :55.

Tversky, A. Kahneman, D. (1981). The framing of decisions and the psychology of choice. *Science,* 211 :453-458.

UKCC, (1991). *The report of the post-registration education and practice project.* London, United Kingdom Central Council.

Uys, L. (1987). Foundational studies in nursing. *Journal of Advanced Nursing,* 12 :275-280.

Vaughan, B. (1990). Knowing that and knowing how: the role of the lecturer-practitioner. In: Salvage, J. Kershaw, B. (eds). *Models for nursing 2.* London, Scutari Press.

Ventura, M.R. Waligora-Serafin, B. (1981). Study priorities identified by nurses in mental health settings. *International Journal of Nursing Studies*, 18 :41-46.

Ventura, M.R. Fox, R.N. Corley, M. Mercurious, S.M. (1982). A patient satisfaction measure as a criterion to evaluate primary nursing. *Nursing Research,* 31 :226-230.

Vinokuv, A (1971). Review and theoretical analysis of the effects of group processes upon individual and group decisions involving risk. *Psychological Bulletin,* 76 :231-250.

Visher, J.S. O'Sullivan, M. (1970). Nurse and patient responses to a study of milieu therapy. *American Journal of Psychiatry,* 127 :451-456.

Von Bertalanffy, L. (1951). General systems theory: a new approach to unity of science. *Human Biology,* 121 :303-361.

Vousden, M. (1986). Removing labels. *Nursing Times,* 82(27) :18-19.

Vousen, M. (1987). Into the community: haven of care... or sick joke? *Nursing Times,* 83(25) :28-30.

Wald, F.S. Leonard, R.C. (1964). Towards development of nursing practice theory. *Nursing Research,* 13(4) :309-313.

Walker F. M. Campbell, S. M. (1989). Pain assessment, nursing models and the nursing process. In Akinsanya, J. (ed) *Theories and models of nursing.* Edinburgh, Churchill Livingstone.

Walsh, M. (1989). Model example. *Nursing Standard,* 22(3) :22-24.

Walsh, M. (1990). From model to care plan. In Salvage, J. Kershaw, B. (eds) *Models for nursing 2.* London, Scutari Press.

Walsh, M. (1991). *Models in clincal nursing: the way forward.* London, Balliere Tindall.

Wandelt, M. Ager, J. (1974). *Quality patient care scale.* New York, Appleton Century Crofts.

Ward, M.F. Bishop, R. (1981). *The quality of acre and the nursing process.* Hellesden Hospital, Norfolk, Unpublished paper.

252

Watson, G. (1973). Resistance to change. In: Zaltman, G. (ed) *Processes and phenomena of social change*. New York, John Wiley & Sons.

Watson, J. (1979). *A model of caring: an alternative health care model for nursing practice and research*. New York, American Nurses Association. (Pub No. NP-593M 8179190).

Weatherston, L. (1979). Theory of nursing: creating effective care. *Journal of Advanced Nursing*, 4 :365-375.

Weaver, T. (1972). The Delphi method: some theoretical considerations. In Ziegler, L.H. Marnen, eds. *The potential of educational futures.*, Worthington, Ohio, Slack publ.

Webb, C. (1984). On the eight day God created the nursing process and nobody rested! *Senior Nurse*, 1(33) :22-25.

Webb, C. ed, (1986). *Using nursing models series: womens health, midwifery and gynaecological nursing*. London, Hodder and Stoughton.

Webb, C. (1986b) Organising care, nursing models: a personal view. *Nursing Practice*, 1 :208-212.

Webb, C. (1991). Action research. In Cormack, D.F.S. (ed) *The research process in nursing*. (2nd ed). Oxford, Blackwell Scientific Publications.

Wells, T. (1980). *Problems in geriatric nursing care*. Edinburgh, Churchill Livingstone.

Whall, A. L. (1989). The influence of logical positivism on nursing practice. *Image*, 21(4) :243-245.

While, A. (1989). *Using a nursing model series: Caring for children: towards partnership with families*. London, Edward Arnold.

White E (1991) A delphi study on psychiatric nursing. *Nursing Times*, 87(32) :48-9.

Whitehead, A.N. (1933). *The aims of education*. London, Benn publications.

Whittingham Hospital Report. (1972). *Report of the committee of inquiry into the Whittingham Hospital*. London, Her Majesty's Stationery Office.

WHSSB, (1990). *Report of a Monitor exercise in a psychiatric hospital*. N. Ireland, WHSSB.

Wiedenbach, E. (1964). *Clinical nursing: a helping art*. New York, Springer Publication Company.

Wilkinson, G. Freeman, H. (1986). *The provision of mental health services in Britain: the way ahead*. London, Gaskell.

Williams, C.A. (1979). The nature and development of conceptual frameworks. In, Downs, F.S Fleming, J.W. eds *Issues in nursing research*. New York, Appleton-Century-Crofts :89-106.

Williams, P. (1974). The district general hospital psychiatric unit and the mental hospital: some comparisons. *British Journal of Prevention of Social Medicine*, 28, :140-145.

Wilson-Barnett, J. (1976). Reflections on progress. *Nursing Times*, 72, :24.

Wilson-Barnett, J. (1978). Patients' emotional response to barium X-rays. *Journal of Advanced Nursing*, 3 :37-46.

Wing, J.K. Brown, C.W. (1961). The social treatment of chronic schizophrenia: a comparative survey of three mental hospitals. *Journal of Mental Science,* 107 :847-861.

Wing, J. (1979). Cited in Meacher, M. ed. *New methods of mental health care.* Oxford, Pergamon Press :209.

Wing, J. (1986). The cycle of planning and evaluation. in Wilkinson, G. Freeman, H. eds. *The provision of mental health services in Britain: the way ahead.* London, Gaskell.

World Health Organisation. (1985). *The principles of quality assurance.* Copenhagen, Euro Reports and Studies (94).

Wright, S.G. (1988). Debate 1. This house believes that nursing models provide a useful tool in the management of patient care. In Pritchard, A.P. (ed) *Proceedings of the 5th International Conference on Cancer Nursing,* London, Macmillan Press.

Wright, S.G. (1986, 1990). *Building and using a model of nursing.* London, Edward Arnold.

Wright, S.G. (1990). Organisational issues of nursing models. *Surgical Nurse,* 3(7) :22-26.

Yoo, K.H. (1991). *Expectation and evaluation of occupational health nursing services, as perceived by occupational health nurses, employees and employers in the United Kingdom.* University of Ulster, Unpublished Ph.D thesis.

Zaltman, G. Duncan, R. (1977). *Strategies for planned change.* New York, John Wiley & Sons.

Zimmer, M.J. (1974). Quality assurance for outcomes of patient care. *Nursing Clinics of North America,* 9(2) :305

# Information note

If the reader wishes to get access to the various research instruments used in this study, or further information about the study itself, they can contact Dr Hugh McKenna at the University of Ulster, N. Ireland direct or they can refer to the dissertation: - McKenna, H.P. (1992). The selection and evaluation of an appropraite nursing model, Unpublished D.Phil thesis, University of Ulster, Coleraine, N. Ireland.